Schizophrenia

Recent Titles in
Q&A Health Guides

Gender Identity and Expression: Your Questions Answered
M. Killian Kinney

Periods: Your Questions Answered
Cristina R. Giambalvo

Healthy Eating: Your Questions Answered
Barbara A. Brehm

Schizophrenia

Your Questions Answered

Romeo Vitelli

BLOOMSBURY ACADEMIC
NEW YORK • LONDON • OXFORD • NEW DELHI • SYDNEY

BLOOMSBURY ACADEMIC
Bloomsbury Publishing Inc, 1385 Broadway, New York, NY 10018, USA
Bloomsbury Publishing Plc, 50 Bedford Square, London, WC1B 3DP, UK
Bloomsbury Publishing Ireland, 29 Earlsfort Terrace, Dublin 2, D02 AY28, Ireland

First published in the United States of America 2025

A catalog record for this book is available from the Library of Congress.

ISBN: HB: 979-8-7651-2032-3
ePDF: 979-8-7651-2034-7
eBook: 979-8-7651-2033-0

Series: Q&A Health Guides

Typeset by Integra Software Services Pvt. Ltd.
Printed and bound in the United States of America

To Peter Li Preti and the Rest of the Shoreham Office
for Their Dedication and Support

Contents

Series Foreword

All of us have questions about our health. Is this normal? Should I be doing something differently? Whom should I talk to about my concerns? And our modern world is full of answers. Thanks to the internet, there's a wealth of information at our fingertips, from forums where people can share their personal experiences to Wikipedia articles to the full text of medical studies. But finding the right information can be an intimidating and difficult task—some sources are written at too high a level, others have been oversimplified, while still others are heavily biased or simply inaccurate.

Q&A Health Guides address the needs of readers who want accurate, concise answers to their health questions, authored by reputable and objective experts, and written in clear and easy-to-understand language. This series focuses on the topics that matter most to young adult readers, including various aspects of physical and emotional well-being as well as other components of a healthy lifestyle. These guides will also serve as a valuable tool for parents, school counselors, and others who may need to answer teens' health questions.

All books in the series follow the same format to make finding information quick and easy. Each volume begins with an essay on health literacy and why it is so important when it comes to gathering and evaluating health information. Next, the top five myths and misconceptions that surround the topic are dispelled. The heart of each guide is a collection of questions and answers, organized thematically. A selection of five case studies provides real-world examples to illuminate key concepts. Rounding out each volume are a directory of resources, glossary, and index. It is our hope that the books in this series will not only provide valuable information but will also help guide readers toward a lifetime of healthy decision-making.

Acknowledgments

Thanks to Maxine Taylor and the diligent Bloomsbury staff for their invaluable aid in completing this book.

Introduction

> *If you are a person with mental illness, the challenge is to find the life that's right for you. But in truth, isn't that the challenge for all of us, mentally ill or not? My good fortune is not that I've recovered from mental illness. I have not, nor will I ever. My good fortune lies in having found my life.*
>
> Elyn R. Saks

In her 2007 memoir, *The Center Cannot Hold*, Elyn Saks, a professor of law and psychiatry at the University of Southern California and recipient of the MacArthur "Genius" Grant, candidly discusses her experiences with schizophrenia. Though she is unsure when her schizophrenia began, she recalls experiencing mild psychotic episodes as early as eight years old. These early episodes, characterized by feelings of unreality and confusion, were a precursor to the more severe symptoms she would face later in life.

As she progressed through college and graduate school, Saks's condition deteriorated. She began to experience more intense and frequent episodes of delusions and paranoia. At times, she would find herself mumbling incoherently, losing track of time, and neglecting basic self-care like eating and bathing. Despite these challenges, Saks was determined to succeed academically and professionally. However, her mental health issues reached a crisis point during her studies at Oxford University and later at Yale Law School, where she experienced her first full-blown psychotic episode.

During these episodes, Saks was forcibly restrained and administered antipsychotic medication against her will. These experiences were traumatic, but they also marked a turning point in her life. Despite the severity of her symptoms, Saks managed to keep her condition hidden from most of her peers and professors. She developed coping mechanisms, such as isolating herself when she felt her symptoms worsening, to maintain some semblance of control over her life. She once explained, "For the most part, I can control what I say, even though I really can't control what I think."

Professor Saks's story is one of resilience and determination. With the support of her husband, Will, and a network of friends, family, and medical professionals, she was able to manage her condition and build a successful career in law and academia. Her achievements are particularly remarkable given the stigma and misunderstandings surrounding schizophrenia and other mental illnesses. Many of her colleagues only became aware of her struggle when she published her memoir, revealing the extent of her battle with schizophrenia.

While Saks's story is inspirational, it also highlights the broader challenges faced by people with schizophrenia. Schizophrenia is a severe mental health condition that impacts millions of people around the world. The World Health Organization estimates that approximately 24 million people live with schizophrenia, though this figure is subject to debate due to differences in diagnosis and reporting across various regions. Regardless of the exact number, it is clear that schizophrenia is a significant public health issue, one that is compounded by the stigma and misconceptions that surround it. This stigma can be particularly debilitating, as it often prevents individuals from seeking the help they need out of fear of being labeled "crazy" or being ostracized by society.

The stigma associated with schizophrenia is one of the most significant barriers to treatment and recovery. Many people with schizophrenia face discrimination not only from the broader society but also within their own families and communities. This discrimination can manifest in various ways, including social isolation, exclusion from employment opportunities, and even mistreatment within healthcare settings. The fear of being judged or rejected often leads individuals with schizophrenia to hide their condition, which can exacerbate their symptoms and make it more challenging to manage their illness effectively.

One of the key challenges in addressing schizophrenia is the fact that it is not a single, uniform condition. Rather, schizophrenia is a spectrum of disorders that can manifest in a variety of ways. People with schizophrenia may experience a range of symptoms, including hallucinations, delusions, disorganized thinking, and impaired social functioning. These symptoms can be incredibly distressing and can significantly impair an individual's ability to function in daily life. However, it is important to note that schizophrenia is not about having multiple personalities or being disconnected from reality by choice. Instead, it involves perceiving the world in a disorienting and frightening way, making it difficult for individuals to distinguish between what is real and what is not.

Understanding schizophrenia requires looking beyond the symptoms to see the person who is living with the condition. It is essential to recognize the humanity of individuals with schizophrenia, to see them as more than just a diagnosis. This understanding is often hindered by widespread myths and misconceptions about the condition. For example, many people falsely associate schizophrenia with violence, despite evidence showing that individuals with schizophrenia are more likely to be victims of violence than perpetrators. This misconception contributes to the stigma that surrounds schizophrenia and can lead to further isolation and discrimination for those living with the condition.

The consequences of this stigma are profound. Social isolation is a common experience for people with schizophrenia, as they may be shunned by friends, family, and colleagues who do not understand their condition. This isolation can lead to feelings of loneliness and despair, which can exacerbate the symptoms of schizophrenia and make it even more difficult for individuals to seek help. In addition to social isolation, people with schizophrenia often face discrimination in the workplace. They may be passed over for job opportunities, denied promotions, or even fired because of their condition. This discrimination can make it challenging for individuals with schizophrenia to achieve financial independence and can contribute to the high rates of poverty and homelessness among people with mental illness.

Another significant consequence of the stigma surrounding schizophrenia is the lack of access to appropriate healthcare. Many people with schizophrenia do not receive the treatment they need because they are too afraid or ashamed to seek help. This can lead to a worsening of symptoms and can increase the risk of hospitalization, homelessness, and even suicide. Addressing and debunking the myths that contribute to this stigma are crucial to creating a more supportive and understanding society.

The perception and treatment of schizophrenia have evolved significantly over time. In the past, schizophrenia was often seen as a moral failing or even as evidence of demonic possession (and still is in many places). People with schizophrenia were frequently subjected to inhumane treatment, including confinement in asylums, where they were often neglected or abused. Over time, however, our understanding of schizophrenia has shifted toward a more compassionate and scientific approach. Advances in psychiatry and neuroscience have shed light on the biological and psychological factors that contribute to schizophrenia, leading to more effective treatments and a greater emphasis on the importance of mental healthcare.

This shift in understanding reflects broader changes in societal attitudes toward mental health. Today, there is a growing recognition of the importance of mental health and the need for comprehensive mental healthcare. However, despite these advances, much work remains to be done to address the stigma and discrimination that people with schizophrenia continue to face. Continued advocacy and education are essential to improving the lives of those living with schizophrenia and to creating a society that is more inclusive and supportive of individuals with mental health conditions.

At the heart of efforts to better understand schizophrenia is the need to dismantle the barriers created by stigma and misinformation. Education and awareness are key to fostering compassion and empathy for individuals with schizophrenia. By recognizing their basic humanity, their dreams, and their potential contributions, we can change the narrative surrounding schizophrenia from one of fear and isolation to one of community and support. This shift in perspective is essential to improving the quality of life for individuals with schizophrenia and to helping them achieve their full potential.

One way to challenge the stigma surrounding schizophrenia is by sharing personal stories and experiences. Books like Elyn Saks's *The Center Cannot Hold* serve as a bridge, connecting the general public to the realities of living with schizophrenia. Her memoir offers a rare and intimate glimpse into the challenges and triumphs of living with the condition, providing valuable insights into the resilience and strength required to manage schizophrenia. Through personal stories like Saks's and the case histories found in this book, we can gain a clearer, more compassionate perspective on schizophrenia and mental illness in general.

Such case histories also remind us that behind every diagnosis is a unique individual with a life full of dreams, challenges, and the potential for joy. While schizophrenia is a chronic condition with no cure, it does not prevent people like Elyn Saks and others from leading rich and rewarding lives with the right treatment and support. These stories challenge the misconceptions and stereotypes that often surround schizophrenia and help to break down the barriers of stigma and discrimination.

As readers, you are invited to approach these stories as opportunities to learn more about schizophrenia and to challenge your own preconceptions about mental illness. With increased understanding comes the power to make a difference—to become advocates for a society that views mental health with the seriousness and empathy it deserves. By educating ourselves and others about the realities of living with schizophrenia, we can help to create a more supportive and inclusive society where individuals with mental health conditions are seen, supported, and valued.

In conclusion, addressing the stigma and misconceptions surrounding schizophrenia is essential to improving the lives of individuals with the condition.

This requires a shift in perspective from seeing schizophrenia as a source of fear and isolation to recognizing it as a condition that can be managed with the right treatment and support. By educating ourselves and others, by challenging our own preconceptions, and by advocating for a more compassionate and inclusive society, we can help to create a world where individuals with schizophrenia are seen, supported, and valued. The stories of individuals like Elyn Saks remind us that while schizophrenia is a challenging condition, it does not define the person who lives with it. With the right support, people with schizophrenia can lead fulfilling and meaningful lives, contributing to society in valuable and important ways.

Guide to Health Literacy

On her thirteenth birthday, Samantha was diagnosed with type 2 diabetes. She consulted her mom and her aunt, both of whom also have type 2 diabetes, and decided to go with their strategy of managing diabetes by taking insulin. As a result of participating in an after-school program at her middle school that focused on health literacy, she learned that she can help manage the level of glucose in her bloodstream by counting her carbohydrate intake, following a diabetic diet, and exercising regularly. But, what exactly should she do? How does she keep track of her carbohydrate intake? What is a diabetic diet? How long should she exercise and what type of exercise should she do? Samantha is a visual learner, so she turned to her favorite source of media, YouTube, to answer these questions. She found videos from individuals around the world sharing their experiences and tips, doctors (or at least people who have "Dr." in their YouTube channel names), government agencies such as the National Institutes of Health, and even video clips from cat lovers who have cats with diabetes. With the guidance of the librarian and the health and science teachers at her school, she assessed the credibility of the information in these videos and even compared their suggestions to some of the print resources that she was able to find at her school library. Now, she knows exactly how to count her carbohydrate intake level, how to prepare and follow a diabetic diet, and how much (and what) exercise is needed daily. She intends to share her findings with her mom and her aunt, and now she wants to create a chart that summarizes what she has learned that she can share with her doctor.

Samantha's experience is not unique. She represents a shift in our society; an individual no longer views himself or herself as a passive recipient of medical care but as an active mediator of his or her own health. However, in this era when any individual can post his or her opinions and experiences with a particular health condition online with just a few clicks or publish a memoir, it is vital that people know how to assess the credibility of health information. Gone are the days when "publishing" health information required intense vetting. The health information landscape is highly saturated, and people have innumerable sources where they can find information about practically any health topic. The sources (whether print, online, or a person) that an individual consults for health information are crucial because the accuracy and trustworthiness of the information can potentially affect his or her overall health. The ability to find, select, assess, and use health information constitutes a type of literacy—health literacy—that everyone must possess.

The Definition and Phases of Health Literacy

One of the most popular definitions for health literacy comes from Ratzan and Parker (2000), who describe health literacy as "the degree to which individuals have the capacity to obtain, process, and understand basic health information and services needed to make appropriate health decisions." Recent research has extrapolated health literacy into health literacy bits, further shedding light on the multiple phases and literacy practices that are embedded within the multifaceted concept of health literacy. Although this research has focused primarily on online health information seeking, these health literacy bits are needed to successfully navigate both print and online sources. There are six phases of health information seeking: (1) Information Need Identification and Question Formulation, (2) Information Search, (3) Information Comprehension, (4) Information Assessment, (5) Information Management, and (6) Information Use.

The first phase is the *information need identification and question formulation* phase. In this phase, one needs to be able to develop and refine a range of questions to frame one's search and understand relevant health terms. In the second phase, *information search*, one has to possess appropriate searching skills, such as using proper keywords and correct spelling in search terms, especially when using search engines and databases. It is also crucial to understand how search engines work (i.e., how search results are derived, what the order of the search results means, how to use the snippets that are provided in the search results list to select websites, and how to determine which listings are ads on a search engine results page). One also has to limit reliance on surface characteristics, such as the design of a website or book (a website or book that appears to have a lot of information or looks aesthetically pleasant does not necessarily mean it has good information) and language used (a website or book that utilizes jargon, the keywords that one used to conduct the search, or the word "information" does not necessarily indicate it will have good information). The next phase is *information comprehension*, whereby one needs to have the ability to read, comprehend, and recall the information (including textual, numerical, and visual content) one has located from the books and/or online resources.

To assess the credibility of health information (*information assessment* phase), one needs to be able to evaluate information for accuracy, evaluate how current the information is (e.g., when a website was last updated or when a book was published), and evaluate the creators of the source—for example, examine site sponsors or type of sites (.com,.gov,.edu, or.org) or the author of a book (practicing doctor, a celebrity doctor, a patient of a specific disease, etc.) to determine the believability of the person/organization providing the information. Such credibility perceptions tend to become generalized, so they must be frequently reexamined (e.g., the belief that a specific news agency always has credible health information needs continuous vetting). One also needs to evaluate the credibility of the medium (e.g., television, internet, radio, social media, and book) and evaluate—not just accept without questioning—others' claims regarding the validity of a site, book, or other specific source of information. At this stage, one has to "make sense of information gathered from diverse sources by identifying misconceptions, main and supporting ideas, conflicting information, point of view, and biases" (American Association of School Librarians [AASL], 2009, p. 13) and conclude which sources/information are valid and accurate by using conscious strategies rather than simply using intuitive judgments or "rules of thumb." This phase is the most challenging segment of health information seeking and serves as a determinant of success (or lack thereof) in the information-seeking process. The following section on Sources of Health Information further explains this phase.

The fifth phase is *information management*, whereby one has to organize information that has been gathered in some manner to ensure easy retrieval and use in the future. The last phase is *information use*, in which one will synthesize information found across various resources, draw conclusions, and locate the answer to his or her original question and/or the content that fulfills the information need. This phase also often involves implementation, such as using the information to solve a health problem; making health-related decisions; identifying and engaging in behaviors that will help a person to avoid health risks; share the health information found with family members and friends who may benefit from it; and advocate more broadly for personal, family, or community health.

The Importance of Health Literacy

The conception of health has moved from a passive view (someone is either well or ill) to one that is more active and process based (someone is working toward preventing or managing disease). Hence, the dominant focus has shifted from doctors and treatments to patients and prevention, resulting in the need to strengthen our ability and confidence (as patients and consumers of healthcare) to look for, assess, understand, manage, share, adapt, and use health-related information. An individual's health literacy level has been found to predict his or her health status better than age, race, educational attainment, employment status, and income level (National Network of Libraries of Medicine, 2013). Greater health literacy also enables individuals to better communicate with healthcare providers such as doctors, nutritionists, and therapists, as they can pose more relevant, informed, and useful questions to healthcare providers. Another added advantage of greater health literacy is better information-seeking skills, not only for health but also in other domains, such as completing assignments for school.

Sources of Health Information: The Good, the Bad, and the In-between

For generations, doctors, nurses, nutritionists, health coaches, and other health professionals have been the trusted sources of health information. Additionally, researchers have found that young adults, when they have health-related questions, typically turn to a family member who has had firsthand experience with a health condition because of their family member's close proximity and because of their past experience with, and trust in, this individual. Expertise should be a core consideration when consulting a person, website, or book for health information. The credentials and background of the person or author and conflicting interests of the author (and his or her organization) must be checked and validated to ensure the likely credibility of the health information they are conveying. While books often have implied credibility because of the peer-review process involved, self-publishing has challenged this credibility, so qualifications of book authors should also be verified. When it comes to health information, currency of the source must also be examined. When examining health information/studies presented, pay attention to the exhaustiveness of research methods utilized to offer recommendations or conclusions. Small and nondiverse sample size is often—but not always—an indication of reduced credibility. Studies that confuse correlation with causation are another potential issue to watch for. Information seekers must also pay attention to the sponsors of the research studies. For example, if a study is sponsored by manufacturers of drug Y and the study recommends that drug Y is the best treatment to manage or cure a disease, this may indicate a lack of objectivity on the part of the researchers.

The internet is rapidly becoming one of the main sources of health information. Online forums, news agencies, personal blogs, social media sites, pharmacy sites, and celebrity "doctors" are all offering medical and health information targeted to various types of people in regard to all types of diseases and symptoms. There are professional journalists, citizen journalists, hoaxers, and people paid to write fake health news on various sites that may appear to have a legitimate domain name and may even have authors who claim to have professional credentials, such as an MD. All these sites *may* offer useful information or information that appears to be useful and relevant; however, much of the information may be debatable and may fall into gray areas that require readers to discern credibility, reliability, and biases.

While broad recognition and acceptance of certain media, institutions, and people often serve as the most popular determining factors to assess credibility of health information among young people, keep in mind that there are legitimate internet sites, databases, and books that publish health information and serve as sources of health information for doctors, other health sites, and members of the public. For example, MedlinePlus (https://medlineplus.gov) has trusted sources on over 975 diseases and conditions and presents the information in easy-to-understand language.

The chart here presents factors to consider when assessing the credibility of health information. However, keep in mind that these factors function only as a guide and require continuous updating to keep abreast of the changes in the landscape of health information, information sources, and technologies.

The chart can serve as a guide; however, approaching a librarian about how one can go about assessing the credibility of both print and online health information is far more effective than using generic checklist-type tools. While librarians are not health experts, they can apply and teach patrons strategies to determine the credibility of health information.

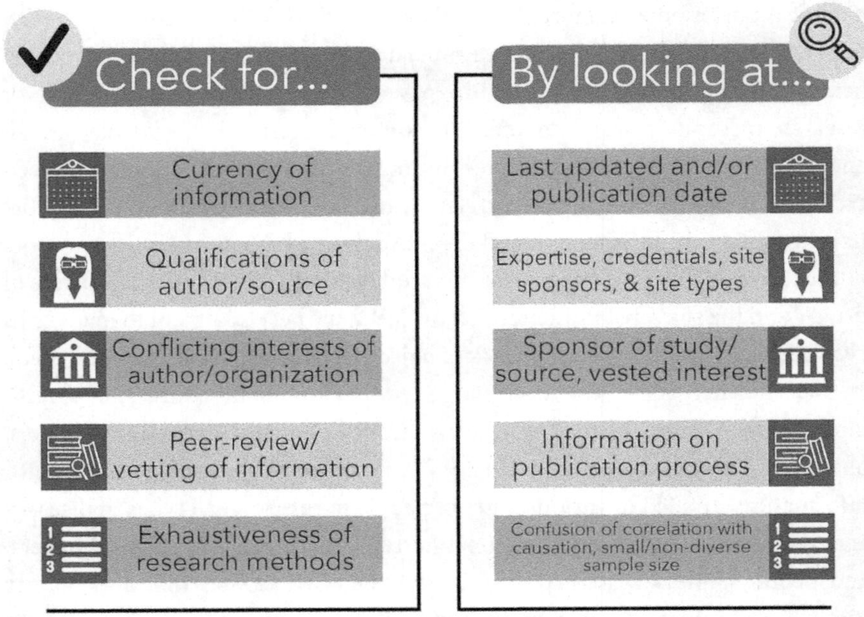

All images from flaticon.com

With the prevalence of fake sites and fake resources that appear to be legitimate, it is important to use the following health information assessment tips to verify the health information that one has obtained (St. Jean et al., 2015, p. 151):

- **Don't assume you are right**: Even when you feel very sure about an answer, keep in mind that the answer may not be correct, and it is important to conduct (further) searches to validate the information.
- **Don't assume you are wrong**: You may actually have correct information, even if the information you encounter does not match—that is, you may be right and the resources that you have found may contain false information.
- **Take an open approach**: Maintain a critical stance by not including your preexisting beliefs as keywords (or letting them influence your choice of keywords) in a search, as this may influence what it is possible to find out.
- **Verify, verify, and verify**: Information found, especially on the internet, needs to be validated, no matter how the information appears on the site (i.e., regardless of the appearance of the site or the quantity of information that is included).

Health literacy comes with experience navigating health information. Professional sources of health information, such as doctors, healthcare providers, and health databases, are still the best, but one also has the power to search for health information and then verify it by consulting with these trusted sources and by using the health information assessment tips and guide shared previously.

Mega Subramaniam, PhD
Associate Professor, College of Information Studies,
University of Maryland

References and Further Reading

American Association of School Librarians (AASL). (2009). *Standards for the 21st-century learner in action.* Chicago, IL: American Association of School Librarians.

Hilligoss, B., & Rieh, S.-Y. (2008). "Developing a unifying framework of credibility assessment: Construct, heuristics, and interaction in context." *Information Processing & Management*, 44(4), 1467–84.

Kuhlthau, C. C. (1988). "Developing a model of the library search process: Cognitive and affective aspects." *Reference Quarterly*, 28(2), 232–42.

National Network of Libraries of Medicine (NNLM). (2013). *Health Literacy.* Bethesda, MD: National Network of Libraries of Medicine. Retrieved from nnlm.gov/outreach/consumer/hlthlit.html.

Ratzan, S. C., & Parker, R. M. (2000). "Introduction." In C. R. Selden, M. Zorn, S. C. Ratzan, & R. M. Parker (Eds.), *National Library of Medicine Current Bibliographies in Medicine: Health literacy*. NLM Pub. No. CBM 2000–1. Bethesda, MD: National Institutes of Health, U.S. Department of Health and Human Services.

St. Jean, B., Subramaniam, M., Taylor, N. G., Follman, R., Kodama, C., & Casciotti, D. (2015). The influence of positive hypothesis testing on youths' online health-related information seeking. *New Library World*, 116(3/4), 136–54.

St. Jean, B., Taylor, N. G., Kodama, C., & Subramaniam, M. (2017). Assessing the health information source perceptions of tweens using card-sorting exercises. *Journal of Information Science.* Retrieved from http://journals.sagepub.com/doi/abs/10.1177/0165551516687728.

Subramaniam, M., St. Jean, B., Taylor, N. G., Kodama, C., Follman, R., & Casciotti, D. (2015). Bit by bit: Using design-based research to improve the health literacy of adolescents. *JMIR Research Protocols*, 4(2), paper e62. Retrieved from http://www.ncbi.nlm.nih.gov/pmc/articles/PMC4464334/.

Valenza, J. (2016). Truth, truthiness, and triangulation: A news literacy toolkit for a "post-truth" world [Web log]. Retrieved from http://blogs.slj.com/neverendingsearch/2016/11/26/truth-truthiness-triangulation-and-the-librarian-way-a-news-literacy-toolkit-for-a-post-truth-world/.

Common Misconceptions about Schizophrenia

1. People with schizophrenia have multiple personalities

The mistaken belief that individuals with schizophrenia possess multiple personalities is a widespread misunderstanding, conflating two separate and distinct psychological conditions: schizophrenia and dissociative identity disorder (DID), formerly known as multiple personality disorder. The misconception stems from a misunderstanding of the term *schizophrenia*, which literally means "split brain" according to the original Latin. What the term means is that schizophrenics experience a "splitting" between their thoughts, emotions, and perceptions, not the multiple personalities reported in DID. Schizophrenia is a complex mental health disorder that can produce a variety of symptoms, including hallucinations, delusions, and disorganized thought processes. These symptoms affect the ability of schizophrenics to interpret how they perceive the world around them, as well as influence their thoughts, emotions, and behaviors. Conversely, DID is characterized by the existence of two or more distinct personality states or identities within a single individual, often as a result of severe trauma. Along with being much rarer than schizophrenia, the DID diagnosis remains controversial and is not classified as a mental illness. See Question 1 for more information.

2. Schizophrenia is a result of poor parenting

While the misconception surrounding "refrigerator parents" and how they can cause mental illness is more commonly associated with autism, it has unfortunately been linked to schizophrenia as well. Not only is this misconception untrue, but it can also inflict guilt on the parents of schizophrenics who face enough of a burden dealing with their children's needs. Modern medical research has amply demonstrated that schizophrenia can be linked to a range of different factors, such as genetic predispositions, neurobiological imbalances, and environmental stressors, rather than because of how children are raised. Still, while family influences can play a role in our mental well-being, these influences are only part of the picture when it comes to schizophrenia. Instead, schizophrenia should be viewed as a biomedical condition rather than something caused by bad parenting or "possession" encourages the development of targeted treatments and support mechanisms, ultimately contributing to improved outcomes for those affected and their loved ones. See Question 9 for more details.

3. Individuals with schizophrenia are dangerous or violent

While movies featuring "mad slashers" such as Norman Bates or Hannibal Lecter may make for gruesome entertainment, they also help perpetuate the stereotype that schizophrenics are inherently dangerous or violent. Such stereotyping is not only potentially dangerous but untrue. Far from being perpetrators of violence, research shows that people grappling with schizophrenia are much more likely to be *victims* of violence rather than the other way around. Not only does this damaging misconception breed unnecessary stigma and fear, but it casts a long, dark shadow over what schizophrenics really experience. Imagine how it would be to deal with the world around you while battling symptoms such as hallucinations and delusions, which can distort your reality and make you feel profoundly alone and misunderstood. By seeing all schizophrenics as being potentially dangerous, far too many people become blind to the actual human beings behind the diagnosis. While schizophrenics need compassion, support, and a deep level of understanding, especially from loved ones, the fear created by misconceptions such as this often undermines how people interact with them. By clinging to and spreading such myths, we do a disservice not only to those with the condition but to the very fabric of our community. See Question 17 for more information.

4. People with schizophrenia have to be institutionalized to get the care they require

The archaic notion that people with schizophrenia need to be tucked away in institutions to manage their condition couldn't be further from the truth today.

Thanks to remarkable advances in mental healthcare, including breakthroughs in medication and the development of comprehensive community support systems, people diagnosed with schizophrenia have the opportunity to experience life in ways that might not have been possible even fifty years ago. Not only can the right treatment help schizophrenics maintain their basic dignity, but they can interact with family, friends, and society as a whole without sacrificing their independence. Imagine the profound difference it makes when a person is supported to integrate socially rather than being isolated—a world where they're seen for fulfilling their potential, not just their symptoms. Sadly, there are far too many schizophrenics who are not getting the care they need and often end up in substandard care, in prisons, or even becoming homeless. Allowing such schizophrenics to be abandoned this way only serves to reinforce harmful stereotypes and create major crises for modern societies around the world. See Question 34 for more information.

5. People with schizophrenia can't lead independent, fulfilling lives

As we've already seen, there are still popular misconceptions about schizophrenia which suggest that people with schizophrenia are somehow incapable of leading normal, fulfilling lives. Misconceptions like that can be extremely harmful to people with schizophrenia and their families, not to mention undermining the support they might receive. They also fail to reflect what many schizophrenics learn to overcome as they navigate life with their symptoms. Due to the amazing progress made in the past few decades, better medications and therapies, along with improved support networks, have made it possible for more schizophrenics than ever to function as a part of society. Today, people with schizophrenia are not only able to excel in academic pursuits, follow successful careers, and maintain deep, lasting relationships but inspire other people dealing with mental illness worldwide. See Questions 5 and 18 for more information.

Questions and Answers

The Basics

1. What is schizophrenia and are there different types?

Despite all the misconceptions surrounding schizophrenia, the reality is that it is a highly complex mental health condition that can manifest itself in many different ways. Not only is schizophrenia a disorder of the mind, but it can also distort how individuals see reality, not to mention having a profound impact on thinking, emotions, and behaviors.

Classified as a major mental illness, schizophrenia makes it almost impossible to distinguish between what is real and what is not. The hallucinations, delusions, and extremely disordered thinking and behavior that schizophrenics experience can dramatically undermine daily functioning unless they get the treatment they need to control these symptoms. As we've already seen, schizophrenia has nothing to do with having a "split personality," such as what people reporting multiple personalities are said to experience. Instead, schizophrenia's hallmark is a fragmented interpretation of reality, making it challenging for sufferers to manage emotions, carry out daily tasks, or conventionally relate to other people.

Usually beginning in late adolescence or early adulthood, schizophrenia symptoms are broadly categorized into *positive*, *negative*, and *cognitive* symptoms. Positive symptoms include hallucinations (seeing or hearing things that are not present) and delusions (false beliefs not based on reality), which add to one's experience of the world in a way that is not based on reality. Negative symptoms involve a diminishing or absence of ability to function normally, such as a lack of motivation, withdrawal from social life, communication difficulties, or diminished emotional expression. Cognitive symptoms involve changes in memory or other aspects of thinking, like trouble focusing or following conversations, which can make everyday tasks challenging.

It is important to recognize that schizophrenia is not a one-size-fits-all condition and can be reflected in different ways. While there are several classic types, each with its own set of symptoms and challenges, the complex nature of schizophrenia can mean that each individual's experiences can be unique. These classic types are:

Paranoid Schizophrenia: Once considered the most common type, individuals with this form primarily experience auditory hallucinations and delusions. For example, they might hear voices that comment on their behavior or converse with each other. They may also have delusions of persecution or grandeur, but their cognitive functions might remain relatively intact.

Disorganized Schizophrenia: This type is characterized by disorganized speech and behavior, as well as flat or inappropriate emotions. Disorganized schizophrenics might have trouble organizing their thoughts or may speak in a way that's hard to understand. They may also exhibit behaviors that don't make sense or are not appropriate to the situation.

Catatonic Schizophrenia: This rare form of schizophrenia involves disturbances in movement. Affected individuals may exhibit motor immobility or excessive, pointless activity. Catatonia can also present with *waxy flexibility*, where an individual's limbs remain in the position they are placed by someone else, e.g., placing an arm in front of the face.

Undifferentiated Schizophrenia: This classification is used when symptoms don't clearly align with the specific types of schizophrenia but the diagnosis of schizophrenia is still appropriate. Individuals might have symptoms across different categories, making it hard to pinpoint a more specific type.

Residual Schizophrenia: In this form, the individual might have a history of acute schizophrenia, but currently has no prominent positive symptoms (such as hallucinations or delusions). They might, however, still display negative symptoms, like withdrawal from social activities or lack of motivation. This is the form of schizophrenia most commonly seen in long-term psychiatric patients.

It's important to note that the Diagnostic and Statistical Manual of Mental Disorders, Fifth Edition (DSM-5) has moved away from these subtypes in favor of a single diagnosis of schizophrenia, recognizing how fluid symptoms can be and their tendency to overlap. Instead, the diagnosis now emphasizes the severity of the symptoms across various dimensions of the illness.

In conclusion, schizophrenia extends beyond the outdated notion of split personality and can fall along a broad spectrum of mental health disorders, many of which can be extremely difficult to diagnose or treat. By understanding the different types of schizophrenia and recognizing the complexity of these different symptoms, we can learn to be more understanding, improve treatment approaches, and ultimately improve the lives of those affected and their families. Through knowledge and compassion, we can dismantle the stigma surrounding this condition and create for a more inclusive and supportive society.

2. How is schizophrenia related to psychosis?

While schizophrenia is a specific mental health condition, psychosis is a symptom that can occur in a range of different mental health disorders. Defined as a condition of the mind that results in difficulty telling what is real from what is not, psychosis can encompass a range of symptoms, including hallucinations and impairments in reality testing. When someone is diagnosed as psychotic, it means that their grasp of the shared reality that guides most of us through our daily lives has slipped, leading to profound disorientation and distress.

On the other hand, schizophrenia, as we've already seen, is a chronic mental health condition characterized by disruptions in thought processes, perceptions, emotional responsiveness, and social interactions. While psychosis is a cornerstone symptom of schizophrenia, often seen as the most visible feature of the disorder, it can occur in many other disorders, some of which we will explore later on.

For those living with schizophrenia, psychosis is not merely a clinical term but a deeply personal reality that undermines how they see and interact with the world around them. To hear voices that no one else can hear or to believe in a reality which others tell you doesn't exist can be intensely frightening, not to mention something that can isolate schizophrenics from those who might provide the love and support they need.

For those dealing with schizophrenia, the experience of psychosis can be particularly jarring, for both schizophrenics themselves and their loved ones. It's a stark reminder of the brain's power to alter perception and the delicate balance required to navigate reality.

But psychosis can occur in other mental health conditions, such as bipolar disorder during extreme manic or depressive episodes or as a result of substance abuse or certain medical conditions. Psychosis can also present itself in different ways, whether as a series of relatively brief phases interspersed with periods of relative clarity, while for others, it may be more constant. The path to managing these experiences is equally varied, often involving a combination of medication, therapy, and support from loved ones and mental health professionals. The different forms psychosis can take highlight the need for careful diagnosis and treatment tailored to the individual's experiences and needs.

In conclusion, while schizophrenia and psychosis are intrinsically linked, their relationship is complex and deeply personal. By approaching this topic with empathy and openness, we can overcome the stigma associated with schizophrenia and psychosis, not to mention encouraging and fostering a more supportive environment for people who are affected. Understanding psychosis within the framework of schizophrenia is not just about recognizing symptoms but about acknowledging how resilient and courageous those who live with these realities are.

3. How common is schizophrenia and is the number of diagnosed cases increasing?

We may never know how many schizophrenics are there worldwide, especially since far too many countries fail to provide reliable statistics. Still, international bodies such as the World Health Organization do what they can to provide an overview of how much of a global health crisis schizophrenia truly is. This condition is estimated to affect about 1 percent of the world's population, a statistic that has remained relatively stable over time despite changes in diagnostic criteria and awareness. This prevalence figure translates into millions of individuals and families navigating the realities of schizophrenia, each with their own unique stories of struggle, resilience, and hope. The stability of schizophrenia's prevalence rate, however, reflects the challenges involved in diagnosing and treating people who are affected, as well as helping them gain greater acceptance.

The question of whether the number of diagnosed cases of schizophrenia is increasing is difficult to answer. On the one hand, advancements in mental health awareness and diagnostic techniques have likely led to more people being accurately diagnosed, particularly in regions and communities where mental health disorders were historically underrecognized. This increased recognition is a positive development since early and accurate diagnosis can significantly improve the quality of life for those with schizophrenia, offering them access to treatments and support systems at an earlier stage.

On the other hand, there have also been improvements in societal attitudes toward mental health. As stigma decreases and understanding increases, more individuals may feel confident enough to seek help for their symptoms, leading to diagnoses that might have been missed otherwise. What this means is that rather than there being a rise in schizophrenia itself, there has been a significant improvement in our society's ability to recognize and address it.

Families and loved ones play a crucial role in the lives of those with schizophrenia, providing support, understanding, and advocacy. Sharing the schizophrenia journey with people who care also makes it easier to manage the complexities of the healthcare system, societal stigma, and the emotional toll of seeing a loved one struggle. These shared experiences demonstrate the importance of community support, mental health education, and resources for both individuals with schizophrenia and their families.

As we consider the prevalence of schizophrenia and the number of diagnosed cases, it's essential to remember that behind every statistic is a person facing daily challenges and success in their journey with this condition. By focusing on the human stories behind the statistics, we can foster a more supportive environment for people affected by schizophrenia, emphasizing the importance of more research, improved treatments, and increased societal acceptance and support.

4. Are certain demographic groups more likely to be diagnosed with schizophrenia?

While schizophrenia does not discriminate when it comes to age, gender, race, or socioeconomic status, there are patterns that suggest certain demographic groups may be more likely to receive a diagnosis. These patterns reflect the basic disparities that contribute to these differences.

Possible reasons for this can include being exposed to stressors such as pollution, noise, and social isolation more intensely than those in rural areas, or simply because people in urban areas are more likely to have access to mental health services and proper diagnosis. Still, this urban-rural divide is very real and can reflect the impact of our living environments on mental health and the need for targeted support and resources in urban communities.

Gender also plays a role in the diagnosis of schizophrenia, with men being far more likely than women to be diagnosed with schizophrenia at a younger age (typically in late adolescence or early adulthood) and may experience more severe symptoms at the onset. Women, on the other hand, may face a later onset, often in their late twenties to early thirties, and their symptoms can sometimes be less pronounced, leading to more difficulty in being properly diagnosed. This gender difference not only affects the experience of those living with schizophrenia but also highlights the importance of gender-sensitive approaches in mental healthcare.

Racial and ethnic disparities in schizophrenia diagnoses are particularly concerning since they can reflect the kind of inequality and bias that can impede effective diagnosis and treatment. Studies have shown that individuals from minority ethnic groups, especially in Western countries, are more likely to be diagnosed with schizophrenia. This finding raises critical questions about the role of cultural differences and racial bias in mental health assessments. Misinterpretations of symptoms, language barriers, and a lack of culturally competent care can all occur, thus leading to misdiagnosis or overdiagnosis in these communities. Problems of this nature underscore the need for a more inclusive approach to mental healthcare.

There can also be socioeconomic factors which affect the likelihood of being diagnosed with schizophrenia. Whether due to reduced access to healthcare, increased exposure to stressors, or a higher probability of experiencing trauma, people from lower socioeconomic backgrounds face an elevated risk of schizophrenia. This association between socioeconomic status and schizophrenia diagnosis demonstrates the need for affordable mental health services for those most vulnerable.

In conclusion, while schizophrenia itself can cross demographic and socioeconomic lines, these patterns in diagnoses remind us that there are broader factors at work which can affect the kind of treatment schizophrenics can receive. There needs to be greater advocacy for mental health equality so that everyone, regardless of their background, has access to the care and support they need. By humanizing our approach to understanding schizophrenia, we can move closer to a world where mental health is recognized and supported with compassion and dignity for all.

5. Are there any famous individuals with schizophrenia?

Schizophrenia can touch the lives of people from all walks of life, including well-known individuals whom you might not realize are dealing with mental health issues. Stories of famous individuals with schizophrenia not only help fight the stigma surrounding this often-misunderstood condition but can also remind us that mental illness does not discriminate by fame, talent, or achievement. These stories help demonstrate how resilience and creativity can help many schizophrenics to succeed in life despite their illness.

One such story is that of John Nash, a brilliant mathematician whose life and battle with schizophrenia were famously depicted in the film *A Beautiful Mind*. Nash's contributions to game theory revolutionized economics and earned him the Nobel Prize in Economic Sciences in 1994. Despite the profound challenges posed by his condition, which became apparent in his early thirties, Nash's story shows his remarkable recovery and profound intellectual achievement. It also underscores the potential for individuals with schizophrenia to lead lives of significant contribution and meaning.

Another individual whose life reflects both the struggle and the potential of living with schizophrenia is Syd Barrett, the founding member of the iconic rock band Pink Floyd. Barrett's innovative guitar work and songwriting helped to define the psychedelic rock genre in the late 1960s. Sadly, his promising career was cut short as he struggled with mental health issues, including symptoms of schizophrenia. Barrett's withdrawal from public life and subsequent solo work inspires fans and artists alike, as a poignant reminder of the delicate balance between creativity and vulnerability.

Then, there is the world of art, which has also seen the brilliance of minds touched by schizophrenia. Louis Wain, an English artist known for his playful drawings of cats, began to exhibit signs of schizophrenia later in his life. His artwork, which grew increasingly abstract and complex as his condition progressed, offers a fascinating window into the mind of someone navigating the realities of schizophrenia. Wain's legacy challenges us to consider the unique perspectives and insights that can accompany mental health conditions, urging a broader appreciation for the diversity of human perception and expression. For that matter, there have been famous artists whose illness has defied clear diagnosis such as Vincent Van Gogh, Edvard Munch, and Camille Claudel who have all been committed in psychiatric asylums for much of their lives yet still managed to enrich the world with their creations.

In the realm of literature, Jack Kerouac, a key figure of the Beat Generation, shared in his writings and letters accounts of his experiences with symptoms akin to those of schizophrenia. Kerouac's groundbreaking work, including his novel *On the Road*, has left an indelible mark on American literature and culture. His life story, marked by both brilliance and struggle, adds to the tapestry of narratives that link creativity and mental health challenges.

All of their stories, while unique in their own way, highlight the mental health challenges they faced and which countless other schizophrenics continue to face every day. We need to recognize their stories as a way of dismantling the stigma surrounding schizophrenia and respect the resilience these stories show and how important it is to look beyond the diagnosis and see the person underneath.

Causes and Risk Factors

6. Do people with schizophrenia have brains that are structured or function differently?

Based on decades of research into the human brain and mental illness itself, the answer to this question is unequivocally "yes." Understanding these differences not only teaches us about the nature of schizophrenia but also helps us move beyond stereotypes to foster empathy and support for people dealing with this condition.

When compared to non-schizophrenics, the brain structure and function in individuals with schizophrenia show distinct variations. While these differences are not uniform across everyone with schizophrenia, they do provide insights into how complex it can be. As new advances in brain imaging are made, such as magnetic resonance imaging (MRI) and positron emission tomography (PET) scans, to name just a few, studies have revealed distinct alterations in brain volume, activity patterns, and connectivity among different brain regions.

One of the most significant findings is the difference in brain volume, i.e., size of the brain as measured by weight, skull volume, or neuroimaging. Studies have consistently shown that individuals with schizophrenia often have reduced volumes in specific brain areas, including the prefrontal cortex and temporal lobes. These regions are critical for cognitive functions such as decision-making, memory, and auditory and visual information processing. The reduction in volume can affect how individuals with schizophrenia perceive reality, leading to symptoms like hallucinations and delusions.

Furthermore, the cerebral ventricles, the four interconnected cavities in the brain, are typically larger in individuals with schizophrenia. Such enlargement may indicate reduced brain tissue, further highlighting structural differences. The significance of these changes is still under investigation, but they suggest a biological underpinning to the symptoms experienced by those with schizophrenia.

Functional differences in the brains of people with schizophrenia have also been documented, particularly in how brain regions communicate and synchronize. For example, there is often altered activity in the default mode network (DMN), a brain network thought to be involved in self-referential thoughts and the resting state. Consisting of the dorsal medial prefrontal cortex, posterior cingulate cortex, precuneus, and angular gyrus, the DFM is most active during activities such as daydreaming or mind-wandering, not to mention whenever we are focused on planning for the future or remembering the past. The alternate DFM activity found in schizophrenics may contribute to the difficulty such individuals may have in distinguishing internal thoughts from external reality, a hallmark of the disorder.

Dysfunction in neurotransmitter systems, particularly those involving dopamine and glutamate, has also been identified. Dopamine is a neuromodulatory molecule that is the most common neurotransmitter in the human body. Along with multiple other roles, dopamine is associated with the brain's reward system and is thought to play a role in the development of psychotic symptoms. Glutamate, the most abundant neurotransmitter, is critical for brain plasticity and learning. Imbalances in these systems can disrupt the brain's normal signaling, leading to the cognitive, emotional, and behavioral symptoms characteristic of schizophrenia.

Although we are only just beginning to understand the complex role that the brain can play in schizophrenia, research into the brain's remarkable plasticity has already resulted in better treatments to manage symptoms and improve the quality of life. As more research expands our understanding of the brain's intricacies, we can expect even newer and more effective treatments in the future.

Understanding the structural and functional differences in the brains of those with schizophrenia is not about labeling; it's about recognizing the biological aspects of a complex condition. We will explore this in more detail later on.

7. What role does genetics play in schizophrenia?

As our understanding of molecular biology and genetics advances, the role human genetics can play in schizophrenia is becoming steadily clearer. Not only does this greater understanding help shed light on schizophrenia's origins but it also offers hope for better treatments and more positive outcomes.

While the link between genetics and schizophrenia is undeniable, it is not as straightforward as we once believed. Studies show that if one identical twin has schizophrenia, the other twin has a 40–50 percent chance of developing the condition, even in different environments. This high rate of concordance in identical twins, who share the same DNA, points to a strong genetic component. However, the fact that the rate is not 100 percent indicates that genetics alone does not determine the development of schizophrenia; there are other factors at work, including environmental and prenatal ones.

The current consensus among researchers is that schizophrenia is a *polygenic* disorder, meaning it's influenced by many different genes, each making a small but important contribution. Researchers have identified more than 100 genetic factors that appear more frequently in people with schizophrenia. These different genes are involved in various crucial processes, such as brain development, neurotransmitter regulation, and immune system function.

The interplay between these genetic factors and environmental influences further complicates the picture. Factors such as prenatal exposure to viruses, malnutrition, or stress, as well as psychosocial stressors like trauma or drug use, can interact with genetic predispositions to increase the risk of developing schizophrenia. This complex interaction between genes and environment highlights the need to move beyond simple cause-and-effect models and to explore better prediction models for diagnosis and treatment.

Understanding the genetic component of schizophrenia is more than an academic pursuit; it has profound implications for individuals and families affected by the condition. For many, knowing that genetics plays a role in schizophrenia can provide a sense of understanding. It can relieve the misplaced guilt or stigma families often feel, wondering if they did something to cause their loved one's illness. Instead, genetics helps us view schizophrenia as a medical condition, influenced by factors largely beyond our control.

Still, this knowledge brings challenges as well. The idea of a genetic predisposition to schizophrenia can raise concerns of what this might mean for future generations. But risk is not destiny, and a genetic predisposition does not guarantee that someone will develop schizophrenia. For that matter, not having any known family members with schizophrenia does not mean that there isn't still a risk.

The ongoing research into the genetics of schizophrenia is paving the way for personalized medicine, where treatments can be tailored to an individual's genetic makeup. This means potentially offering more effective and less intrusive treatment options and allowing for earlier identification and intervention for those at higher genetic risk. The end result will be greater understanding and empathy, better support, and improved hope for the future.

8. How do prenatal factors influence the risk of schizophrenia?

Prenatal factors, including fetal development and environmental exposures during pregnancy, play a crucial role in determining the risk of developing schizophrenia later in life. Understanding these factors emphasizes the profound impact of our early development on mental health later in life. Among these factors are nutritional deficiencies, exposure to toxins or infections, and maternal stress during pregnancy.

Studies have shown that malnutrition, particularly during early pregnancy, can increase the risk of schizophrenia in offspring. This is thought to be due to the essential role of nutrients in brain development. For example, deficiency in folic acid, a vital nutrient for DNA synthesis and repair, has been linked to an increased risk of schizophrenia, emphasizing the importance of adequate maternal nutrition for brain health.

Exposure to infections during pregnancy is another prenatal factor associated with an increased risk of schizophrenia. Viral infections like influenza, rubella, and toxoplasmosis, when contracted by the mother during pregnancy, can impact fetal brain development in unexpected ways. The immune response to these infections, including the production of inflammatory cytokines, is thought to affect the developing brain and potentially predispose the child to schizophrenia, especially if there is a preexisting family history of the disease.

Maternal stress is also a significant prenatal factor. High levels of stress experienced by the mother during pregnancy can influence the development of the fetal brain. The release of stress hormones, such as cortisol, can cross the placenta and affect the fetus, potentially leading to alterations in brain development that increase the risk of schizophrenia. This highlights the importance of supporting mental and emotional well-being during pregnancy.

Moreover, prenatal exposure to toxins, such as alcohol, drugs, or environmental pollutants, can have a profound impact on fetal brain development. These substances can interfere with normal brain growth processes, increasing the likelihood of schizophrenia and other developmental disorders.

The impact of these prenatal factors on the risk of schizophrenia underscores the critical importance of prenatal care and environmental conditions. It also challenges us to think more broadly about mental health, recognizing that the foundations for our mental well-being might be laid long before we are born. By understanding and addressing these prenatal factors, we can begin to take steps toward preventing schizophrenia and other mental health conditions.

In conclusion, the prenatal period is a window of opportunity for influencing the long-term mental health of individuals. The risk of schizophrenia, influenced by a complex interplay of genetics and environmental factors, can be markedly affected by prenatal conditions. By prioritizing prenatal care and supporting mothers, society can make strides in reducing the likelihood of schizophrenia and improving the lives of those affected by it.

9. Which environmental factors may contribute to schizophrenia?

As we have seen, while genetics play a critical role in the risk of developing schizophrenia, environmental factors also significantly contribute to its onset. These factors can be broadly categorized into prenatal exposures, childhood experiences, and adult life circumstances. As we have seen in the previous section, prenatal factors, including fetal development and parenting exposures during pregnancy, play a crucial role in determining the risk of developing schizophrenia later in life. However, childhood is also a critical period for brain development, making environmental factors particularly influential during this development period.

Traumatic experiences, such as physical or emotional abuse, neglect, or loss of a parent, can increase the risk of developing schizophrenia later in life. These early-life stressors can disrupt the normal development of the brain's stress response systems, potentially leading to the onset of schizophrenia in genetically predisposed individuals. And the role such environmental factors can play factors in schizophrenia extends into adulthood as well.

According to numerous studies, stress, drug use, and urban living can also be significant contributors to schizophrenia. Chronic stress, whether from personal relationships, financial difficulties, or other sources, can exacerbate or trigger schizophrenia in susceptible individuals. The use of psychoactive drugs, particularly cannabis, has been shown to increase the risk of different forms of psychosis, including schizophrenia, especially in those with a genetic predisposition to these conditions. Additionally, living in an urban environment has been linked to a higher incidence of schizophrenia, suggesting that the complexity and stressors associated with urban life may play a role in its development.

It's important to note that the impact of environmental factors on schizophrenia is not isolated; instead, it interacts with genetic predispositions in a dynamic interplay. This means that while environmental factors can increase the risk of schizophrenia, their effects are often moderated by an individual's genetic makeup. Understanding this interaction is key to developing personalized treatment and prevention strategies.

Discussing the environmental factors contributing to schizophrenia is not about assigning blame or oversimplifying a complex condition. Instead, it's about fostering empathy, reducing stigma, and supporting those affected by the disorder. By acknowledging the role of environmental factors, we recognize the profound impact of our surroundings on our mental health. This understanding encourages a more compassionate view of schizophrenia, highlighting the importance of supportive communities, early intervention, and comprehensive care.

In conclusion, the environmental factors contributing to schizophrenia underscore its complexity and the need for a better understanding of mental health. Recognizing how these factors impact the likelihood of developing serious mental illness also promotes a more supportive approach to those living with schizophrenia. It's a call to action for society to address the environmental risks that can lead to mental health disorders and to ensure that individuals have access to the care and support they need to live fulfilling lives.

10. Can substance abuse trigger schizophrenia?

While substance abuse does not directly cause schizophrenia, research suggests it can trigger psychosis, and even full-blown schizophrenia, in those who are genetically predisposed to developing psychotic symptoms. This distinction is crucial in understanding the interplay between substance use and mental health, and it underscores the importance of addressing substance abuse not just for its immediate effects but also for its potential to precipitate severe psychiatric conditions in vulnerable individuals.

While the onset of schizophrenia is typically in late adolescence or early adulthood, a period coincidentally associated with increased rates of substance use, psychoactive drugs like cannabis, stimulants, and hallucinogens (e.g., LSD) can often worsen psychotic symptoms in individuals predisposed to schizophrenia. Cannabis is the most widely studied substance in this context. Research suggests that heavy and prolonged use, especially of high-potency strains, can increase the risk of developing schizophrenia-like psychosis. This is particularly true for individuals with a family history of the disorder or those who have experienced early-life trauma, indicating a complex interaction between genetic vulnerability, environmental stressors, and substance use.

Explaining why substance abuse might trigger schizophrenia suggests an interplay of neurobiological factors and the individual's genetic makeup. Psychoactive substances can alter brain chemistry and neural pathways, potentially worsening or triggering underlying psychiatric conditions. For susceptible individuals, this can mean an earlier onset of schizophrenia or the intensification of its symptoms, leading to an earlier and more severe disease course.

Understanding this relationship is not only a research issue; it has profound implications for prevention and treatment. It also highlights the importance of early intervention and targeted support for at-risk youth, particularly those with a family history of schizophrenia or early signs of mental health issues. Substance abuse prevention and treatment programs for people who are at increased risk for psychosis can play a critical role in mitigating the risk of schizophrenia.

As we have seen, while substance abuse alone does not cause schizophrenia, it can trigger schizophrenia's onset in those already predisposed to the disorder. This relationship underscores the importance of a holistic approach to mental health, considering the interplay of genetic, environmental, and lifestyle factors. We can better support those at risk as we learn more about these complex interactions. This not only addresses the individual needs of those affected by substance abuse and schizophrenia but can also have a dramatic impact on the healthcare costs associated with treating this frustrating disease.

11. Can schizophrenia be prevented?

The question of whether schizophrenia can be prevented is one that resonates deeply within the medical community, among families, and across society. Given the damage schizophrenia can have on individual sufferers and their families, the potential for prevention is a topic of great interest and importance. While there is no definitive answer that guarantees prevention, current research and understanding suggest pathways that may reduce the risk or delay the onset of schizophrenia.

One of the most promising approaches in the quest to prevent schizophrenia or lessen its impact is early detection and intervention. Identifying individuals at high risk for developing schizophrenia—such as those with a family history of the disorder or who have experienced early warning signs like mild, transient psychotic symptoms—can be crucial. Early intervention programs that provide psychological support, education, and in some cases, medication, can potentially delay or even prevent the onset of full-blown schizophrenia in some individuals.

As we have already discussed, certain prenatal factors, such as exposure to infections, malnutrition, or extreme stress during pregnancy, can increase the risk of a child developing schizophrenia later in life. Thus, improving prenatal care and support for expectant mothers, ensuring access to adequate nutrition, and reducing their exposure to stress and infection can be important preventive measures. These efforts underscore the importance of maternal and fetal healthcare as a component of schizophrenia prevention strategies.

We have also seen that substance abuse, particularly in adolescence and young adulthood, is linked to an increased risk of developing schizophrenia, especially in those with a family history of the disorder. Public health initiatives aimed at reducing substance abuse, including education about the risks associated with drug use, particularly psychoactive and hallucinogenic drugs, can play a significant role in prevention efforts.

Along with the other environmental influences we have examined, psychosocial factors in the development of schizophrenia are also being recognized. Childhood trauma, social isolation, and chronic stress can all increase the risk of developing schizophrenia, especially in combination with genetic influences. This is why promoting social cohesion, support networks, and stress management skills from a young age can help boost resilience and potentially reduce the risk of developing schizophrenia.

Despite these strategies, it's important to approach the subject of prevention with sensitivity and care. For individuals and families affected by schizophrenia, the suggestion that the condition could have been prevented may carry implications of blame or regret. Prevention in the context of schizophrenia does not justify blame; instead, it stresses how important it is to understand the complex factors contributing to the condition.

In conclusion, while there is no surefire way to prevent schizophrenia, early detection, prenatal care, substance abuse treatment, and emphasizing overall well-being may reduce the risk or delay the onset of the disease. As our understanding of schizophrenia continues to evolve, so too will our strategies for prevention, offering hope and support to those affected by the condition and their families.

Features of Schizophrenia

12. What are hallucinations?

Hallucinations, a phenomenon often shrouded in mystery and misunderstanding, are perceptions without external stimuli. Vivid sensations of sight, sound, smell, taste, or touch can trick people into believing they are perceiving something that isn't actually there. Far from being a mere figment of the imagination or a whimsical daydream, hallucinations are complex experiences that can have a profound impact on those who experience them.

At their core, hallucinations challenge our understanding of how we interpret the world around us. The human brain is an extraordinary organ that constantly processes sensory information to navigate our environment. However, under certain conditions, this intricate system can become disrupted, leading to perceptions without external cues. These experiences can be as mundane as feeling your phone vibrate when it hasn't or as vivid and complex as seeing and interacting with people or entities that are not there.

While there are many medical conditions which can produce hallucinations, along with those produced by certain substances (e.g., LSD or cannabis), or even loss of sleep or extreme thirst, the hallucinations resulting from mental health conditions such as schizophrenia can be particularly distressing. Individuals dealing with schizophrenic episodes can hear voices making critical comments or commanding them to perform actions (known as command delusions), and they can often experience a profound sense of isolation from the world around them.

People experiencing such hallucinations for the first time in their lives are especially vulnerable to feelings of confusion, fear, and a sense of losing control. For others, they may be benign or even comforting, such as the sound of a lost loved one's voice. The subjective nature of these experiences makes them deeply personal, affecting each individual in unique ways.

In recent years, research into the mechanisms behind hallucinations has offered insights into how they occur, paving the way for better treatments and interventions. This scientific exploration underscores the importance of approaching hallucinations with curiosity and compassion, seeking to understand rather than to judge. While hallucinations are far more common than most people realize, they need to be taken seriously whenever they occur, given how important they can be in diagnosing and treating diseases.

13. What are delusions?

Delusions are among the most misunderstood and fascinating aspects of human psychology. They represent a profound distortion of reality, where the affected person holds strong beliefs in things that are not true or highly exaggerated despite evidence. Unlike simple misbeliefs that can be corrected with new information, delusions are rigid and persist even when faced with clear evidence that contradicts them. Understanding delusions requires us to delve into the complexities of the human mind, recognizing the delicate balance between perception, belief, and reality.

Delusions can take different forms, each reflecting a unique disturbance in the individual's understanding of the world. Some may believe in grandiose scenarios where they possess extraordinary powers or wealth. In contrast, others may be convinced of a conspiracy against them (or the world in general) and feel persecuted by unseen forces or individuals. There are also *delusions of reference*, where mundane occurrences are believed to have significant personal meanings, and *somatic delusions*, involving a preoccupation with health and organ function. Each type of delusion can seem undeniably real to the individual and often paints a vivid picture of the brain's capacity to create intricate scenarios that make perfect sense. At least, at first.

The experience of living with delusions can be isolating and terrifying. Imagine the distress of being convinced that loved ones are impostors (Capgras syndrome) or the new people you meet are actually familiar people in disguise (Fregoli syndrome). For that matter, imagine feeling as if you are actually dead or otherwise didn't exist (Cotard's syndrome). These are not mere quirks of thought but profound disruptions in the ability to discern reality, often leading to significant impairment in social and occupational functioning. Individuals rarely choose to believe these things on their own; instead, their brain is presenting them with a distorted version of reality that is as convincing to them as the real world is to us.

While delusions are most commonly associated with psychiatric disorders such as schizophrenia, severe depression, and bipolar disorder, they can also occur in the context of neurological conditions or as a result of substance misuse. This means that a comprehensive approach to diagnosis and treatment is vital in understanding when someone develops such delusions. Only by understanding the underlying cause can we address these delusions effectively.

In conclusion, delusions challenge our understanding of reality and belief, highlighting the brain's incredible power to shape how we perceive the world. By learning more about delusions, we can provide better support for people who experience them and find more effective ways of treating them as they occur.

14. What is disorganized thinking and speech?

Disorganized thinking and speech are symptoms often associated with certain mental health conditions, most notably schizophrenia, but also in other disorders. Such disorganized speech goes beyond the occasional stumble in our words or momentary mind-wandering that everyone experiences. It represents a more profound disruption in communicating coherent thoughts effectively. Understanding how disorganized thinking and speech affect schizophrenics demonstrates its profound impact on their ability to connect with others and navigate daily life.

At its core, disorganized thinking means being unable to organize thoughts in a logical sequence. This can result in a disjointed flow of ideas, making it hard for the individual to maintain a focused conversation or complete tasks that require structured thought processes. For someone experiencing disorganized thinking, the world can feel like a jigsaw puzzle where the pieces don't quite fit together. Thoughts may jump from one topic to another without apparent connection, or they may become stuck in a loop, repeating the same idea without progression.

Disorganized speech, also known as thought disorder, is the outward manifestation of disorganized thinking. It involves speech that is difficult to follow, with abrupt changes in topic, illogical sequencing of ideas, or the use of made-up words and phrases. For the listener, it can be challenging to discern the intended message, leading to misunderstandings and frustration on both sides. For the individual, the inability to communicate effectively can be isolating, often resulting in withdrawal from social interactions to avoid embarrassment or confusion.

This disorganization of thought and speech is not simply a matter of "not thinking before speaking." It's a reflection of an underlying disruption in cognitive processes that are essential for organizing and expressing thoughts. This can significantly impact an individual's ability to function in social, academic, and work settings, where clear communication and logical thinking are often crucial. One example of a formal thought disorder which can occur in schizophrenia is *circumstantiality*, or the use of "labyrinthine" speech that includes numerous trivial, and often senseless, additional details that seem to make sense to the schizophrenic but are thoroughly confusing to people with whom they are communicating. Another example is tangential speech, involving a loss of focus, so schizophrenics can often "wander off" verbally without ever returning to their original topic.

To understand why disorganized thinking and speech can occur in schizophrenia, we need to look at the different genetic, neurological, and environmental factors which research has already narrowed down to abnormalities in certain brain regions involved in thought processing and language, including the brain's right hemisphere. Understanding these underlying mechanisms is key to developing effective treatments and support strategies for helping people with formal thought disorders. Healthcare professionals trained to help such patients can often get through by using simple strategies when the patient's words don't make sense. These include asking clarifying questions, avoiding assumptions, and giving the person time to express their thoughts.

Cognitive-behavioral therapy (CBT) and other forms of psychotherapy can also help individuals develop strategies to organize their thoughts and improve their communication skills along with better medications.

In conclusion, disorganized thinking and speech deeply affect individuals' ability to communicate and connect with the world around them. Recognizing these symptoms and the distress they can cause is vital in providing effective treatment and help schizophrenics access the resources they need to live fulfilling lives.

15. How can schizophrenia affect movement and motor behavior?

While schizophrenia is usually considered to be a major mental illness, it can also have a serious impact on body movement and motor behavior. This reflects how complex schizophrenia can be and how it might touch every aspect of a schizophrenic's life.

Movement problems in schizophrenia can take many different forms and range from very subtle signs that might only be noticeable to trained health professionals to far more serious problems such as catatonia, stereotyped movements, or motor agitation (all of which we will discuss.)

Catatonia, for example, is one of the most striking ways in which schizophrenia can affect movement. Individuals experiencing catatonia may find themselves in a state where they are virtually immobile, remaining in the same position for hours or even days. People experiencing catatonia can also display what is known as *waxy flexibility*, which allows a patient's catatonic body to be "posed" as if it were made of wax. This means an arm stretched into a certain position would remain that way until moved. Catatonic symptoms can be extremely distressing, not only for the person experiencing it but also for their loved ones. In other instances, catatonia can manifest as excessive and pointless motor activity that is not influenced by external stimuli. These symptoms starkly illustrate the profound disconnect that can occur between the mind and body in schizophrenia.

Similarly, some individuals with schizophrenia exhibit *stereotyped movements*, which are repetitive, aimless movements that serve no purpose, such as rocking back and forth or tapping a foot incessantly. These behaviors can be misunderstood by those not familiar with the condition, potentially leading to social isolation or stigma.

Motor agitation is another way in which schizophrenia can influence movement, characterized by an inability to sit still and a compulsion to move about constantly. This restlessness can be exhausting for the individual, making it difficult to concentrate or engage in tasks requiring sustained attention.

Beyond these more noticeable effects, schizophrenia can also subtly influence coordination and motor control. Individuals may experience clumsiness, awkward gait, or uncoordinated movements, affecting their ability to perform everyday tasks and diminishing their quality of life.

Understanding the motor symptoms of schizophrenia means recognizing the challenges faced by those who experience them. These motor symptoms can be extremely frustrating since they can affect how well schizophrenics can engage in work, social activities, and even simple daily routines. Addressing these motor symptoms of schizophrenia requires comprehensive treatment, combining medication, physical therapy, and psychosocial support. Though antipsychotic medications can be effective in managing some of the motor symptoms, they can also cause motor problems, whether as a short-term side effect or due to long-term use. This is why such medications need to be carefully monitored to ensure that problems don't arise. Physical therapy and exercise can also improve motor function and overall physical health, while supportive counseling can help individuals cope with the emotional and social challenges accompanying these symptoms.

As we can see, the impact of schizophrenia on movement and motor behavior is a vivid reminder of the need for treatment that can address the full range of symptoms schizophrenics can experience. Teaching patients how to handle these motor symptoms is crucial in providing comprehensive care that truly meets the needs of individuals with schizophrenia.

16. What are other common "negative" symptoms of schizophrenia?

As we have already discussed, *negative symptoms* often seen in schizophrenia involve a loss of normal functions as opposed to *positive symptoms* such as hallucinations and delusions. Understanding negative symptoms can be crucial for providing better care and support to people living with schizophrenia.

Part of the difficulty in dealing with negative symptoms of schizophrenia is how insidious they can be. Though they may not appear at first the way that positive symptoms can, negative symptoms often become more apparent in people who have been suffering from schizophrenia for years. Such negative symptoms can include:

Affective flattening or diminished emotional expression. Individuals displaying this kind of flattening may have a reduced ability to show emotions through facial expressions, voice tone, or body language. This can make it challenging for them to connect socially with others since they can no longer show social cues such as outward signs of joy, sorrow, or affection.

Alogia, or poverty of speech, refers to a reduction in the amount of speech schizophrenics produce as well as the kind of ideas such speech can convey. Conversations with someone experiencing alogia might feel strained, with brief, unelaborated responses that make deep communication difficult. This can further isolate people socially since even simple conversation can become a hurdle.

Anhedonia is the loss of pleasure in activities once enjoyed. Imagine all those activities you once enjoyed suddenly turning dull and unappealing, for example. For individuals experiencing anhedonia, the motivation to engage in these activities dissipates, leading to a life that can feel empty and joyless. Though anhedonia can occur in many mental disorders, especially depression, schizophrenics seem especially vulnerable and, in many cases, can be misdiagnosed as depressed, which would delay proper treatment.

Avolition refers to a lack of motivation or ability to initiate and persist in goal-directed activities. People experiencing avolition can have problems performing everyday tasks, from personal hygiene to pursuing educational or work-related goals. Not only can this be incredibly frustrating, both for schizophrenics and for their loved ones, but, much like anhedonia, can lead to them being misdiagnosed with a mood disorder such as depression.

As with avolition and anhedonia, *social withdrawal* is another common negative symptom which can be misdiagnosed as resulting from depression. Defined as the tendency to retreat from social interactions and relationships, social withdrawal, along with other negative symptoms can often lead to chronic schizophrenics isolating themselves, thus exacerbating the loneliness and misunderstanding that often accompany schizophrenia.

The impact of these negative symptoms extends far beyond the individual and affects families, friends, and communities as well. They can hinder education, employment, and the ability to live independently, leading to the stigma and social isolation associated with schizophrenia.

Unfortunately, while antipsychotic medications can be effective in managing positive symptoms, they are often less effective against negative symptoms, highlighting the need for alternative approaches. Psychotherapy can help individuals develop coping strategies and improve social skills, while social support, including from family, friends, and peer groups, can provide a vital network of understanding and acceptance.

As we see, recognizing and addressing the negative symptoms of schizophrenia can provide better support to those in need. As our knowledge and awareness of these symptoms grow, so too does our capacity to offer hope and help to they affect.

17. Are people with schizophrenia violent?

The stereotype that people with schizophrenia are inherently violent is a pervasive and harmful misconception that promotes the social isolation and discrimination faced by schizophrenics and their families. As we have already seen, the association between schizophrenia and violence is largely exaggerated, with the vast majority of people with schizophrenia being more likely to be victims of violence than perpetrators. Despite high-profile media coverage when looking at rare incidents of violence and schizophrenia, not to mention how people with mental disorders are portrayed in horror movies and television, the reality is very different.

Whatever risk of violence there may be in schizophrenics is typically linked to other factors such as lack of access to treatment, or having a history of violence even before the onset of the illness. It's important to note that these factors are also associated with increased risk of violence in the general population. Substance abuse, in particular, significantly elevates the risk of violent behavior across all groups, not just among those with schizophrenia.

For that matter, personality factors linked to criminal behavior and violence, including psychopathy, can often begin in early childhood, while schizophrenia typically begins much later in life. If someone already had a propensity toward violence or criminal behavior before developing schizophrenia, that risk will only become greater but it will not be the schizophrenic symptoms causing it. But the same can be said of any other mental disorder as well.

Stigmatizing people with schizophrenia as dangerous not only makes them more isolated but can also discourage people experiencing symptoms for the first time from seeking help due to fear of being judged or ostracized. This can lead to worsening symptoms and a far greater likelihood of crisis situations, which, in turn, can be seen as confirming the stereotype. Breaking down this stigma requires public education, advocacy, and a shift in media representation to focus on the *reality* of living with schizophrenia, rather than sensationalizing rare incidents.

By trying to understand schizophrenia, rather than just dwelling on stereotypes, we can better understand the challenges that schizophrenics can face and provide the support they need to function in society.

18. Do people with schizophrenia experience symptoms all the time?

The experience of schizophrenia varies widely among those affected by it making its progress over time hard to predict. Still, much like mood disorders such as depression and bipolar disorder, schizophrenia often follows a cyclical pattern. While there are typically periods of acute psychosis where symptoms are more pronounced (especially in the early stages), they are interspersed with periods of relative stability where symptoms may subside or become less intense. During these stable periods, some individuals might experience a significant reduction in symptoms, allowing them to be more involved in daily activities, relationships, and work. Even during these stable periods, however, negative symptoms can be present which would have a strong impact on overall quality of life and functioning.

The fluctuation of symptoms is influenced by various factors, including whether schizophrenics are adhering to treatment, stress levels, substance use, and the presence of supportive relationships and environments. Adherence to treatment plans can be a particular problem since many schizophrenics refuse to take medication or participate in psychotherapy because they are bothered by side effects or refuse to recognize that their symptoms need treatment. Also, finding the right treatment can be a complex and ongoing process so it can take time to reduce the severity and frequency of acute psychotic episodes significantly.

Understanding the episodic nature of schizophrenia can challenge how society perceives schizophrenics, especially with the stigma surrounding the condition. Individuals with schizophrenia can have periods where they can lead regular lives, despite the difficulty in predicting how their symptoms can fluctuate. For this reason, schizophrenics and their families often develop strategies to manage symptoms and recognize early warning signs of an impending episode.

Support from mental health professionals, peers, and loved ones plays a crucial role in this ongoing process, offering stability and understanding in the face of challenges. Recognizing the variable nature of their symptoms can make schizophrenics easier to treat and avoid the kind of crises that can reinforce traditional stereotypes.

19. How does schizophrenia affect communication and social interaction?

Given that the ability to communicate and form social interactions is a critical part of human connection and understanding, it's not hard to recognize that individuals living with schizophrenia often experience profound isolation due to problems with communicating socially with others. For schizophrenics, symptoms such as disorganized thinking can make it difficult to form coherent thoughts and express them clearly. Conversations may become challenging, with speech patterns becoming tangential or derailed by loosely associated ideas. This can make it hard for others to follow the conversation, leading to frustration on both sides.

Schizophrenia can also affect verbal expression and the ability to interpret social cues. We have already discussed alogia, or poverty of speech, which can often stifle social conversations. Additionally, difficulties in interpreting facial expressions, body language, and other non-verbal signals can further complicate social interactions. This can result in misunderstandings and a sense of disconnection, as individuals with schizophrenia might misinterpret others' intentions or fail to convey their own emotions and responses effectively.

However, schizophrenics can also experience social withdrawal and isolation due to the stress they face because of miscommunicating, along with the fear of being judged by others. Over time, this withdrawal can become a self-fulfilling cycle, worsening feelings of loneliness and isolation. When you consider the negative symptoms of schizophrenia, such as lack of motivation and inability to feel pleasure, it's hardly surprising that they also make schizophrenics more withdrawn. This resulting isolation impacts the individual's quality of life and their support network, as friends and family may feel at a loss for how to maintain connection and support.

Increased empathy from friends, family, and even society at large can make a significant difference in the lives of those affected by schizophrenia. Breaking down the stigma that surrounds schizophrenia is crucial, as it can encourage individuals to seek the help and support they need without fear of judgment. Better education about schizophrenia can help foster a more inclusive and supportive environment in personal relationships and broader societal contexts.

This is why support for individuals with schizophrenia involves more than just medical treatment; it also requires helping them improve their communication skills and social interaction. Therapeutic approaches, such as social skills training and CBT, can provide individuals with strategies to navigate social situations more effectively. Additionally, peer support groups offer a safe space for individuals to connect with others who understand their experiences, fostering a sense of community and belonging.

Understanding the challenges involved in helping schizophrenics overcome social isolation and relationship problems requires a compassionate approach that considers the individual's needs, strengths, and experiences. Through better support and more inclusive communities, we can help people with schizophrenia promote a sense of connection and belonging that enriches their lives and the lives of those around them.

20. How does schizophrenia affect a person's ability to form and maintain relationships?

As we have just seen, schizophrenia can undermine social functioning, often fraying the connections that bind us to one another. This goes well beyond the symptoms themselves but can create barriers in communication. Since schizophrenics often experience disorganized thoughts and speech, conveying ideas and feelings to others becomes much harder. Misunderstandings during conversations can then lead to frustration for schizophrenics as well as their loved ones. Given how important support from friends and family can be, this sense of isolation often makes things worse for schizophrenics, even when their symptoms are under control.

Moreover, the positive symptoms of schizophrenia, such as hallucinations and delusions, can also complicate social interactions. These symptoms can have a dramatic impact of a schizophrenic's sense of reality and make it harder for them to engage in meaningful conversations and social activities as a result. For example, a person who is experiencing delusions of persecution might misinterpret a friend's actions as hostile, even when they are not. This misunderstanding can lead to mistrust and withdrawal, straining or even severing relationships completely.

Then, there are the negative symptoms of schizophrenia, such as emotional flatness and lack of motivation. These symptoms can make it seem like the person is emotionally unavailable or disinterested, leaving friends and family feeling hurt or powerless to help. As schizophrenics appear more withdrawn and apathetic, it can create a gulf between them and their loved ones, further isolating them from the support they need.

Social withdrawal is commonly seen in people struggling with schizophrenia. Given their fear of being judged or misunderstood, schizophrenics often shy away from social interactions to avoid potential hurt or embarrassment. This self-imposed isolation not only removes the support that can help them function, but it also reinforces the stigma surrounding schizophrenia.

While maintaining relationships is often harder with schizophrenics, any challenges can be overcome through good communication, empathy, and informed support. Education about schizophrenia can help friends and family understand schizophrenia's impact and develop strategies to maintain open lines of communication.

Support groups and therapy can provide safe spaces for people with schizophrenia to explore their feelings and learn new ways of interacting with others. Friends and family members can also benefit from support and education, whether through individual counseling or support groups where they can share their experiences with other people who have faced similar challenges.

In summary, while schizophrenia presents significant challenges to forming and maintaining relationships, these challenges are not insurmountable. With understanding, support, and informed strategies, individuals with schizophrenia and their loved ones can build strong relationships with empathy and support and make the challenges faced by schizophrenics a little easier to overcome.

21. How does schizophrenia affect emotions?

Along with hallucinations, delusions, and disorganized thinking, schizophrenia also has a powerful influence on emotions, often in ways that aren't visible but are still deeply felt. Understanding the emotional effects of schizophrenia is crucial in appreciating the full scope of the condition and providing better support to those who live with it.

One of the most striking ways schizophrenia affects emotions is through *blunted* or *flattened affect*, affecting how those emotions are expressed. Individuals with schizophrenia may appear emotionally numb or indifferent, displaying little facial expression or vocal inflection, even in situations that would typically evoke strong emotions. This blunting of affect can be misconstrued as a lack of feeling or detachment from others, but it is important to recognize that it is a symptom of the condition, not a reflection of the schizophrenic's capacity for emotion.

As we've already seen, schizophrenia can also cause anhedonia, the diminished ability to experience pleasure from activities usually found enjoyable. Much as in mood disorders such as depression, this symptom can make it challenging for individuals to engage in social activities, hobbies, or other interests that once brought them joy. This loss of pleasure often contributes to the social withdrawal many schizophrenics display, since losing this incentive to engage in pleasurable activities tends to isolate them further from supportive relationships and enjoyable experiences.

Schizophrenics can also display emotional volatility, causing them to be unpredictable or unable to control their emotions. These sudden emotional shifts, which seem disconnected from external circumstances, can often be distressing and confusing, making it difficult to cope in social situations or maintain personal relationships. The fear of unexpected emotional reactions can add another layer of isolation, as individuals may withdraw in an attempt to manage their emotional responses in private.

Additionally, the cognitive symptoms of schizophrenia, such as disorganized thinking, can make it harder for individuals to understand their own emotions or empathize with others. This can lead to misunderstandings and conflicts in relationships, as intentions and responses may be misinterpreted by both the schizophrenics and those around them.

Supporting someone with schizophrenia involves recognizing how their emotions are part of the broader clinical picture and providing the support they need without judgment. This support can come in many forms, including therapy, medication management, and social support from family, friends, and peer groups. Therapeutic approaches that focus on emotional awareness, expression, and regulation can be particularly beneficial, helping individuals navigate their emotional landscapes more effectively.

By understanding and acknowledging the emotional effects of schizophrenia, we can offer more effective support to those who live with this condition. Fostering better understanding and acceptance is essential in ensuring that schizophrenics do not face these emotional problems alone.

22. How does schizophrenia affect a person's ability to learn and work?

Given that schizophrenia can significantly impact how people think, feel, and behave, it's easy to see how this can create substantial hurdles in pursuing educational and career goals. Understanding these challenges is crucial for meeting the unique needs of schizophrenics and allowing them to achieve goals that might otherwise be denied them.

Certainly, the cognitive symptoms of schizophrenia, including the role they play in memory, attending, and decision-making, will directly affect learning and work performance. These symptoms can also make it challenging for schizophrenics to absorb new information and apply it in practical contexts. For instance, a student with schizophrenia might struggle to follow lectures or complete assignments on time due to problems with focusing or organizing their thoughts. Similarly, an employee with schizophrenia may find it hard to stay on task, meet deadlines, or make quick decisions, even in a familiar job setting.

Then there is the disorganized thinking commonly seen in schizophrenia. Disorganized thoughts can make it more difficult to structure ideas, not to mention cause problems in expressing oneself clearly and coherently. Effective communication is vital to success, whether educationally or in the workplace, and dealing with the challenges resulting from schizophrenia will make it harder to convey their ideas to peers and supervisors, leading to misunderstandings and frustrations.

The negative symptoms of schizophrenia, such as apathy and lack of motivation, can also undermine the ability to succeed with their studies or work. For example, a lack of motivation can make it hard for a person to start tasks, follow through on commitments, or seek out opportunities for advancement. Social withdrawal can make it more difficult for individuals to form supportive relationships that can shape academic and professional development.

Furthermore, the stigma associated with schizophrenia can create barriers in educational and work environments. Misconceptions and biases may lead to discrimination or exclusion, preventing individuals from accessing the same opportunities as their peers. This stigma can discourage individuals from seeking the accommodations or support they need, for fear of being labeled or misunderstood.

Despite these challenges, individuals with schizophrenia can and do succeed in learning and working environments, especially with appropriate support and accommodations. We have already seen cases of people who have managed to succeed in many walks of life despite their schizophrenia.

But the key to getting ahead lies in creating more inclusive environments that recognize and accommodate the unique needs of people with schizophrenia. This can include encouraging educational institutions and workplaces to offer flexible scheduling, better access to quiet workspaces, allowing extra time for tasks, and ensuring access to mental health support services. There are also assistive technologies, such as organizational apps or software designed to improve focus and memory, which can be invaluable tools for people with schizophrenia. Moreover, vocational rehabilitation programs can offer tailored support, helping individuals develop job skills, find suitable employment, and navigate workplace challenges.

While schizophrenia can present challenges for people in educational and work settings, these challenges can still be overcome with understanding, support, and appropriate from employers and co-workers. Creating more inclusive and supportive environments in schools and workplaces is not just beneficial for individuals with schizophrenia, embracing diversity and fostering resilience can create better opportunities and a more positive environment for everyone.

23. Why do individuals with schizophrenia often withdraw from others?

People with schizophrenia often find themselves retreating from social interactions and relationships due to the many difficulties they face in connecting with others. The overwhelming social challenges that schizophrenics face can be overcome by empathy and greater understanding from others, the stigma faced by those with schizophrenia often leads to their becoming more isolated and neglected instead.

Admittedly, the symptoms experienced by many schizophrenics can intimidate many people who lack the proper training to help them cope. Hallucinations and delusions, for instance, can make social interactions confusing and often frightening. Imagine trying to engage in a conversation while simultaneously hearing voices that no one else can or feeling perpetually watched by unseen forces. Helping schizophrenics work through these symptoms is often exhausting, even for friends and family members. As a result, far too many schizophrenics might prefer to isolate themselves as a way of cutting themselves off from those whom they feel don't understand what they are experiencing.

Then there are the negative symptoms such as apathy, anhedonia, and avolition, which can make schizophrenics abandon pleasurable activities or relationships simply because it seems easier to live that way and avoid the distress of trying to be more open with others. Since schizophrenia can also cause difficulties with concentration, memory, and executive functioning, even something as basic as following conversations, interpreting social cues, or expressing thoughts can seem impossible. Faced with these obstacles, social withdrawal can appear as a protective measure against potential embarrassment or the fear of being misunderstood or judged by others.

When you consider the stigma surrounding mental illness, particularly schizophrenia, it's probably not surprising that far too many people "write off" those they deem to be "crazy" and isolate them from potential sources of support and understanding. People with mental illness can internalize this stigma and develop feelings of shame. These feelings can make it even harder for them to reach out for fear of rejection or burdening others. This vicious cycle of stigma and withdrawal underscores how important it is to change how we perceive and respond to mental illness.

Still, withdrawal does not have to be inevitable for those living with schizophrenia. There are certainly numerous treatment alternatives which can help schizophrenics overcome their social withdrawal. Peer support groups can allow individuals to share experiences and strategies with others dealing with schizophrenia. Similarly, family therapy and education can equip loved ones with the tools to support their family member, fostering a nurturing environment that encourages social engagement.

In conclusion, far too many people with schizophrenia prefer to isolate themselves due to their symptoms and the stigma they often face. However, it is possible to help those with schizophrenia develop better social skills and relationships through mental healthcare and education. By bridging the gap between isolation and connection, people with schizophrenia can overcome isolation and lead more social lives.

24. Why do some individuals with schizophrenia self-harm?

Self-harm among individuals with schizophrenia is a deeply concerning issue. Whether it involves cutting themselves, head-banging, punching walls, etc., such behavior is often a distressing sign of the inner turmoil they are experiencing. Understanding why self-harm occurs in people with schizophrenia requires a compassionate approach that acknowledges their symptoms and emotional pain, not to mention how they are coping with their distress. This understanding is crucial for providing effective support and understanding the root causes of self-harm.

One of the primary reasons individuals with schizophrenia self-harm is as a coping mechanism to deal with overwhelming symptoms. Hallucinations and delusions can cause tremendous fear and confusion for those affected. Paradoxically, self-harm can often help manage these feelings by providing a temporary sense of control or a way to distract from the mental anguish caused by psychosis. Since the physical pain of self-harm might momentarily overshadow the psychological pain, it can offer fleeting relief, making it a method they might come to rely on in future.

Furthermore, the negative symptoms of schizophrenia, such as emotional numbness and being unable to feel pleasure or motivation, can also contribute to feelings empty and disconnected. When faced with such symptoms, self-harm becomes a way of feeling when they feel detached from themselves and the world around them.

For that matter, cognitive impairments associated with schizophrenia, including difficulties with executive functioning and decision-making, can affect the ability of many schizophrenics to find healthier coping mechanisms.

This can lead to impulsive behaviors like self-harm without fully understanding the long-term medical and psychological repercussions.

The stigma surrounding schizophrenia can often reinforce feelings of isolation and despair felt by many people and make them more self-destructive as a result.

It is also important to consider the role of other conditions, such as depression or substance use disorders, which can also be experienced by those with schizophrenia. These conditions can independently increase the risk of self-harm, and when combined with the symptoms of schizophrenia, this risk becomes greater.

Mental health professionals, families, and caregivers dealing with schizophrenia needed to accept the greater risk of self-harm schizophrenics can face. Since many self-harming individuals, whether schizophrenic or not, are often afraid to admit what is happening, it is essential that those dealing with them make them feel safe enough to talk about self-harm without the fear of judgment.

In conjunction with effective medications, psychotherapeutic approaches, such as CBT and dialectical behavior therapy (DBT), can be particularly effective in teaching individuals healthier coping strategies, and better ways to manage distressing symptoms. Peer support groups can also offer a space for sharing experiences and strategies, reducing feelings of isolation by connecting with others who understand the challenges of living with schizophrenia.

As we have seen here, self-harm among individuals with schizophrenia is often seen as a way of coping with distressing symptoms, feelings of emptiness, and societal stigma. Understanding *why* self-harm can occur in schizophrenics is vital for developing compassionate and effective treatments. Through comprehensive care and compassion, it is possible to help individuals find healthier ways to cope with their emotions and work for a more positive future.

25. Does schizophrenia tend to co-occur with other conditions?

Schizophrenia does not always exist in isolation but can occur with other conditions, a phenomenon known as comorbidity. The presence of additional disorders alongside schizophrenia can complicate how symptoms can be diagnosed and treated while underscoring the need for a broader approach to care.

One of the most common comorbidities observed in individuals with schizophrenia is substance use disorders, including alcohol, drug, and nicotine dependence. There can be multiple reasons for this. Not only many people may develop substance dependence long before developing schizophrenic symptoms, but some people in the early stages of schizophrenia may turn to substances as a way of self-medicating distressing symptoms of schizophrenia, such as hallucinations and anxiety. Even after receiving treatment, it isn't uncommon for some schizophrenics to turn to drugs or alcohol to mitigate the side effects of antipsychotic medications. However, substance use can exacerbate symptoms of schizophrenia, leading to a worsening of the condition and complicating treatment efforts, not to mention leading to potentially deadly drug interactions. This cycle of substance use and increased psychiatric symptoms requires a combined treatment approach to deal with both the substance use disorder and schizophrenia at the same time.

Depression is another condition frequently found alongside schizophrenia. The overlapping symptoms of these conditions, such as social withdrawal and diminished motivation, can often lead to misdiagnosis, especially in the early stages of schizophrenia. The impact of depression on individuals with schizophrenia can be profound, significantly affecting their quality of life and increasing the risk of suicide. Treatment strategies must, therefore, be designed to address the symptoms of both conditions, often involving a combination of medication, psychotherapy, and social support.

Anxiety disorders, including generalized anxiety disorder, social anxiety disorder, and panic disorder, also frequently co-occur with schizophrenia. The pervasive sense of dread in many anxiety disorders can heighten the unease and paranoia that individuals with schizophrenia may already experience and make them even more isolated than before. Managing anxiety in the context of schizophrenia requires careful treatment with an emphasis on therapies that promote relaxation, stress management, and coping skills.

Additionally, physical health conditions are more common among individuals with schizophrenia, including cardiovascular diseases, diabetes, and respiratory diseases. This is often due to lifestyle factors associated with a chronic mental health condition, such as reduced physical activity and poor diet, but also due to the side effects of some antipsychotic medications. Integrating physical healthcare with psychiatric care is essential for addressing these health disparities and improving the quality of the patients' lives.

Effective treatment plans for schizophrenics must consider the full range of their health needs, including medication management, psychotherapy, lifestyle interventions, and support for substance use disorders. Moreover, comorbidity issues underscore the need for routine screening for additional conditions in individuals diagnosed with schizophrenia, ensuring that all aspects of their health are addressed.

Recognizing and addressing the comorbidities linked to schizophrenia are crucial for improving outcomes and the quality of life. Integrated, personalized care helps manage the complexities of schizophrenia and its comorbid conditions, fostering resilience and hope for those affected.

Diagnosing and Managing Schizophrenia

26. How is schizophrenia diagnosed?

Diagnosing schizophrenia is not an easy process considering that the symptoms, which may first appear at any point from adolescence to late adulthood (but usually in the late teens or early twenties), can often be misdiagnosed when first seen. Diagnosis should only be attempted by a duly qualified healthcare professional with the necessary training and experience for dealing with schizophrenia.

The first step in diagnosing schizophrenia is to gather a comprehensive history of the person's symptoms. Even for someone presenting with many of the positive, negative, and cognitive symptoms of schizophrenia, they aren't enough on which to base a diagnosis. This is because of the significant overlap such symptoms can have with other mental health disorders.

The first step in dealing with a potentially schizophrenic patient is a detailed interview. Mental health professionals, such as psychiatrists or clinical psychologists, conduct these interviews by asking about medical history, symptoms, and personal experiences. During these interviews, patients are encouraged to speak openly about what they're going through, including any hallucinations they are experiencing, beliefs they hold, or changes in their thinking and behavior. This dialogue is essential for understanding the unique symptoms that each person can show.

In addition to the interview, diagnosing schizophrenia usually requires ruling out other potential causes of the symptoms. This could involve a series of medical tests to exclude physical health issues that might mimic or contribute to the symptoms, such as brain tumors, certain vitamin deficiencies, or substance use disorders. Blood tests, imaging studies like MRI or CT scans, and screenings for drugs and alcohol are part of this exclusion process. It involves basic detective work to piece together clues from various angles to arrive at the correct diagnosis.

Another crucial aspect is assessing the duration and impact of symptoms. For a diagnosis of schizophrenia, symptoms must be present for at least six months—and they must significantly impair the individual's ability to function in daily life, i.e., work or school. This prolonged observation period is needed to ensure that the diagnosis is accurate and to provide the right treatment.

Since schizophrenia can often be confused with other mental health conditions, such as bipolar disorder or severe depression with psychotic features, getting the diagnosis right is crucial since the wrong treatment might do more harm than good. As a result, the diagnosis of schizophrenia isn't made lightly and should only be reached through careful consideration and collaboration between healthcare professionals and the person being treated. The process is as much an art as a science, demanding sensitivity, patience, and expertise from those involved.

Once a diagnosis is made, it opens the door to treatment and support tailored to the individual's specific needs and experiences. The aim is to manage symptoms, improve the quality of life, and support the person in achieving their personal goals, whether building relationships, pursuing education or employment, or simply enjoying day-to-day life.

And the diagnosis isn't something written in stone, either. Not only can symptoms change over time, but many schizophrenics develop additional mental health and physical health issues due to the chronic nature of the disease. Whether it is substance abuse to manage symptoms or depression over how schizophrenia is affecting their lives, mental health professionals and family members need to recognize these new problems as they arise.

In essence, diagnosing schizophrenia typically requires combining medical expertise with a deeply human touch. It's about not just looking at the symptoms but also the person behind them to understand their experiences and how they are shaping their mental health.

27. Why is it important to diagnose schizophrenia early?

The importance of diagnosing schizophrenia early cannot be overstated, primarily because it is vital that treatment begins before the condition has the chance to firmly disrupt the life of the individual, not to mention their friends and family. Early intervention programs have been shown to improve outcomes for people with schizophrenia significantly. These programs address symptoms more effectively and help maintain their relationships, educational pursuits, and career aspirations. Essentially, early intervention provides guidance to keep individuals from drifting too far from the life they had planned for themselves.

Early intervention in schizophrenia includes a range of therapeutic and support services designed to address the unique challenges faced by individuals with the disorder. These programs focus on:

1. **Symptom Management**: Early intervention can lead to better control of symptoms such as hallucinations, delusions, and disorganized thinking. Addressing these symptoms early can prevent them from becoming entrenched and more difficult to manage over time.
2. **Support Systems**: Programs that encourage family support have been shown to decrease rehospitalization rates and improve social outcomes. Family members learn how to support their loved ones effectively, creating a more stable and understanding home environment.
3. **Educational and Career Support**: By intervening early, individuals can receive support to continue their education or maintain employment. This support helps them stay connected to their goals and aspirations, reducing the disorder's impact on their future prospects.

Unfortunately, many people in the early stages of schizophrenia may choose to hide their symptoms to avoid being labeled as "crazy" or dangerous. This stigma leads to underreporting and delayed diagnosis. Common early symptoms include visual or auditory hallucinations, delusions, paranoia, or social withdrawal, to name just a few. Depending on how severe the symptoms are and how successful early schizophrenics are at hiding them, proper diagnosis can be delayed for years and make treatment much harder than it needs to be.

People who manage to conceal their schizophrenia are vulnerable to various problems, including disrupted personal and family relationships, substance abuse, unemployment, and homelessness. Early intervention can help avoid these problems by providing diagnosed individuals with the skills and support needed to manage their symptoms and build resilience through therapy, medication, and community support.

Diagnosing schizophrenia early can demystify the condition for the individual and their loved ones. For most people, what they know about schizophrenia is based on stigma and misinformation perpetuated by popular media. Mental health professionals can help individuals and their families replace fear and misunderstanding with accurate information. By encouraging open conversations and sharing experiences, individuals with schizophrenia and their loved ones learn how to move forward with their lives in a constructive and informed manner.

On a societal level, early diagnosis of schizophrenia underscores the importance of mental health awareness and the need for accessible mental health services. By advocating for early recognition and response to symptoms of schizophrenia, society can ensure that people in need receive the mental healthcare they deserve. This proactive approach can reduce the overall burden of the disorder on the healthcare system and improve the quality of life for individuals and their families.

In conclusion, the early diagnosis of schizophrenia is critical for effective treatment and improved long-term outcomes. By addressing symptoms early, providing robust support systems, and educating individuals and their families, we can significantly improve the lives of those affected by schizophrenia. Early intervention benefits the individual and has far-reaching positive effects on their loved ones and society as a whole.

28. Are there other conditions that can be mistaken for schizophrenia or vice versa?

As we've already seen diagnosing schizophrenia can be extremely difficult since it shares symptoms with a variety of other mental health disorders. Understanding these overlaps not only demonstrates how complex mental health problems can be but also emphasizes the importance of thorough, personalized assessments in making an accurate diagnosis.

While schizophrenia is the most common diagnosis when facing symptoms such as hallucinations, delusions, disorganized thinking, and emotional flatness, there are other possible diagnoses which need to be considered. They include:

Bipolar Disorder: Along with its manic highs and depressive lows, bipolar disorder can also introduce hallucinations or delusions, strikingly similar to the psychotic symptoms seen in schizophrenia. However, these symptoms in bipolar disorder are typically *mood-congruent*, meaning they are consistent with the individual's extreme mood (either manic or depressive). The distinction is subtle but crucial, as it influences the approach to treatment and support. Differentiating between schizophrenia and bipolar is particularly essential when it comes to treatment with psychiatric medications, which are very different for the two conditions. Not only can misdiagnosis delay effective treatment, but being prescribed the wrong medication can introduce new medical problems due to side effects.

Major Depressive Disorder with Psychotic Features: Individuals suffering from severe depression may experience psychotic symptoms, such as hallucinations or delusions. These symptoms, however, are generally aligned with the theme of their depression, creating a distinguishable pattern that, with careful evaluation, can be differentiated from the broader range of psychotic symptoms seen in schizophrenia. Again, as with bipolar disorder, it is vital to make a proper diagnosis to ensure that treatment begins as soon as possible and that patients are not given the wrong medications.

Schizoaffective Disorder blurs the lines between schizophrenia and mood disorders even further since it can embody symptoms from both categories. The key to differentiating schizoaffective disorder from schizophrenia lies in the presence of mood disorder symptoms *alongside* psychotic episodes. In schizophrenia, on the other hand, psychotic symptoms are not exclusively tied to mood episodes which can be an extremely subtle distinction to make.

Borderline/Schizoid/Schizotypal Personality Disorder: Although not classified as major mental illnesses, *personality disorders* are basically long-lasting, disruptive patterns of thinking, behavior, mood, or social functioning which can cause long-term adjustment problems for many people. Of the ten personality disorders formally recognized by the Diagnostic and Statistical Manual of Mental Illness (DSM-5), there are three which are most likely to be confused with schizophrenia. Individuals with borderline personality disorder (BPD) may experience brief psychotic episodes under stress, yet these episodes are transient and context-specific, unlike the more enduring psychotic symptoms of schizophrenia. BPD is characterized by a long-term pattern of relationship instability, intense emotional responses, and a distorted sense of self. People with BPD can also experience issues with dissociation (detachment from reality), a fear of abandonment, and paranoia. Schizotypal personality disorder (SPD) is often much harder to differentiate from schizophrenia since it can be characterized by transient psychosis, bizarre beliefs, paranoia, and related symptoms. Schizoid personality disorder (ScPD) can be characterized by emotional coldness, a lack of interest in social relationships, detachment, and apathy. For that matter, it is also possible to be diagnosed with mixed personality disorder, which combines features from two or more of the classic personality disorders. Since the roots of personality disorder can date back to childhood or early adolescence, the onset of personality disorder symptoms typically begin much earlier than with schizophrenia though, as symptoms worsen over time, differentiating personality disorder from mental illness can become much harder as well.

Delusional Disorder involves strong beliefs in things that are not real or true but don't typically feature the full spectrum of psychotic symptoms found in schizophrenia, i.e., hallucinations. Its singular focus on delusions can lead to misinterpretation as schizophrenia, underscoring the importance of making an accurate diagnosis.

Furthermore, *substance-induced psychotic disorders* can mimic schizophrenia, with certain drugs (such as amphetamines or hallucinogens) inducing psychotic symptoms. Distinguishing these substance-induced conditions from schizophrenia requires careful examination of the individual's substance use history and the timing of symptoms. While detox treatment usually results in rapid improvement, this isn't always the case, especially for people who are already at risk for psychosis or who have been taking the substances as a form of self-medication.

The overlap in symptoms among these conditions highlights the critical need for comprehensive, individualized assessments to ensure that the correct diagnosis is made. Mental health professionals often rely on detailed histories, careful observation, and a process of elimination to ensure that patients are correctly diagnosed.

In understanding these potential misdiagnoses, we're reminded of the interplay between various mental health conditions, the importance of thorough assessments, and the profound impact of accurate diagnosis on an individual's path to recovery. Through careful evaluation and a deep commitment to personalized care, we can ensure that individuals receive the support and treatment that truly align with their unique experiences, offering hope and clarity in the journey toward wellness.

29. Can schizophrenia be cured?

For people diagnosed with schizophrenia, not to mention their friends and family, there is the inevitable question of whether a true cure is possible. Seeing loved ones experiencing profound disruptions in thinking, feeling, and behaving, not to mention hearing voices that others do not hear, seeing things that others don't, or believing in realities that are not shared by others, is always heart-breaking so the hope for a cure will always be there. Sadly, as of this book's writing, there is no known cure for schizophrenia in the sense of a complete eradication of symptoms and a return to a pre-disease state. The complex causes of schizophrenia, combining genetics, brain chemistry, and environmental factors, mean that there are no simple answers and no way of eradicating such a chronic condition.

However, the absence of a cure does not equate to a lack of hope or possibilities. The fields of psychiatry and psychology have made significant strides in making schizophrenia much more manageable for many. Through a combination of medication, psychotherapy, and support systems, individuals with schizophrenia can function in the community and avoid the life-long isolation that once characterized this condition.

Medications, particularly antipsychotics, serve as a cornerstone in this management, helping to reduce the intensity and frequency of psychotic symptoms. While finding the right medication to help schizophrenics cope often requires a period of trial and error, many of the newer medications being used help manage symptoms more effectively with much fewer side effects.

Psychotherapy, including individual and group therapies, can be effective in helping people with schizophrenia to explore their thoughts and feelings, to learn strategies for dealing with symptoms, and to connect with others facing similar problems. Therapy sessions can also provide safe spaces where schizophrenics and their loved ones can learn to work together while overcoming the barriers created by misunderstandings and stigma.

Support systems play a critical role in treatment, offering not just a safety net but a way of teaching individuals to explore their abilities, hopes, and relationships. Families, friends, and mental health professionals form a community of care to overcome the isolation that far too many schizophrenics face.

While schizophrenia cannot be "cured" as such, it is possible to help schizophrenics manage their symptoms and improve the quality of their lives. As the dialogue on schizophrenia and its treatment continues to evolve, advances in research, treatment, and societal understanding are providing better opportunities for individuals with schizophrenia to find a more hopeful future together.

30. What medications are used to manage schizophrenia?

While not a cure, medications can still play a crucial role in managing symptoms of schizophrenia while offering individuals a way to get their lives under control. As newer and more effective medications become available, they can offer a beacon of hope for those navigating the challenges of this complex condition.

While antipsychotic medications form the cornerstone of treatment for schizophrenia, they are not one-size-fits-all. These medications are divided into two main groups: first-generation (or typical) antipsychotics and second-generation (or atypical) antipsychotics.

First-generation Antipsychotics have a long history in the treatment of schizophrenia. These medications, including haloperidol, chlorpromazine, and fluphenazine, work by acting on dopamine receptors in the brain. *Dopamine*, a neurotransmitter involved in mood, motivation, and pleasure, is thought to be in excess in certain brain regions in schizophrenia. By blocking its action, these medications can significantly reduce the intensity of psychotic symptoms. However, their performance comes at a cost, often bringing a suite of side effects such as drowsiness, dizziness, and, more notably, *extrapyramidal symptoms* (EPS) affecting movement and muscle control.

Second-generation Antipsychotics offer a different approach. Medications like risperidone, olanzapine, quetiapine, and aripiprazole not only affect dopamine receptors but also affect serotonin, another neurotransmitter implicated in schizophrenia. This broader mechanism of action tends to offer improved efficacy in managing not just the psychotic symptoms but also the emotional and cognitive disturbances that accompany schizophrenia. They come with their own set of potential side effects, such as weight gain and increased risk of diabetes, yet often present a reduced risk of movement disorders compared to their first-generation counterparts.

The choice between these antipsychotics is deeply personal and tailored to the individual's specific symptoms, medical history, and medication side effect profiles. Deciding which medication to use often depends on the individuals and their healthcare providers as they weigh the benefits and risks involved.

In addition to antipsychotics, other medications may also play supporting roles in the management of schizophrenia. *Mood stabilizers* and *antidepressants* may be prescribed to address the mood symptoms that can accompany schizophrenia, while *benzodiazepines* may be used short term to manage acute anxiety or agitation. This ensemble of medications, each with its part to play, comes together to provide a more comprehensive approach to treatment, addressing the myriad ways in which schizophrenia can affect an individual's life.

As we've discussed previously, finding the right medication often involves trial and adaptation since the effects of the medications can vary widely among individuals. Although the process can sometimes be frustrating while searching for the right dosage or medications the benefits outweigh the side effects soon enough, making the symptoms more manageable. This then allows individuals with schizophrenia to get their lives under control and investigate other treatment options such as psychotherapy.

31. What are some possible side effects of the medications used to treat schizophrenia?

When dealing with powerful antipsychotic medications, the relief from distressing symptoms often comes intertwined with potential side effects. These medications, invaluable as they are in treating symptoms of schizophrenia, can carry numerous possible side effects, and each person's experience is as unique as their fingerprint. Learning about these possible side effects is an essential part of the education people with schizophrenia need to receive to understand what to expect as they are being treated. The type of side effects can vary depending on what kind of medication is being prescribed.

We have already discussed first-generation antipsychotics which can be extremely effective in relieving psychosis. Unfortunately, their use in patients is often shadowed by a constellation of side effects known as EPS. These include *dystonia* (painful muscle spasms), *akathisia* (restlessness), and *parkinsonism* (characterized by tremors, stiffness, and movement slowing). While these symptoms are largely manageable, first-generation antipsychotics can also lead to more serious conditions such as *tardive dyskinesia*, a condition marked by involuntary movements, a reminder of the medication's presence long after the day's dose, and even *neuroleptic malignant syndrome*, which can be life-threatening if the medication is stopped immediately.

Due to the risks associated with first-generation antipsychotics, most psychiatrists prefer to prescribe second-generation antipsychotics instead. Unfortunately, while these medications have fewer side effects, they can present different challenges. Weight gain stands out as a common side effect, which can lead to related issues such as diabetes and heart disease. There's also the risk of metabolic syndrome, a gathering storm of conditions that include increased blood pressure, high blood sugar, and abnormal cholesterol levels, each a potential harbinger of more severe health concerns. Additionally, some individuals may experience sedation, which can lower awareness of the world around them, or akathisia, leading to a perpetual restless sensation.

Both classes of antipsychotics can also introduce less serious side effects such as dry mouth, blurred vision, or constipation. Sexual dysfunction and menstrual changes also occur. While not life-threatening, these side effects can still affect daily well-being and undermine mental wellness.

It's essential to remember that many individuals consider these side effects manageable or minimal. However, finding the right medication balance and learning to live with potential side effects shouldn't be faced alone. Support systems, whether in the form of healthcare providers, family, or support groups, provide guidance, understanding, and strategies to manage or mitigate these side effects. Lifestyle changes can also help, whether it involves dietary adjustments to combat weight gain or physical activities to counter sedation.

Learning to cope with side effects is an unavoidable part of the treatment process for individuals with schizophrenia and, for most patients, is not a major concern. How severe those side effects can be will depend on the type of medication being taken, the necessary dosage, and whether people on those medications get the support they need, both from professionals and loved ones.

32. What non-drug therapies and interventions can help individuals with schizophrenia?

While medication serves as a major component of schizophrenia treatment, non-drug therapies and interventions are also essential. Examples of non-drug treatments include:

Psychotherapy, or talk therapy, typically begins once a schizophrenic's initial symptoms are stabilized and they are able to participate in treatment. Cognitive Behavioral Therapy (CBT) represents one of the most effective talk therapies and focuses on teaching participants to manage symptoms by changing thought patterns and behaviors. Along with helping schizophrenics to build a toolkit of strategies to reduce the impact of symptoms, CBT can also teach ways to cope with the stress that often accompanies these symptoms. Different types of CBT can be used, whether individually or in treatment groups, and we will cover these different types later.

Family Therapy is designed to foster understanding and communication within families. By strengthening the emotional support that schizophrenics receive from their loved ones, family therapy is another way of teaching better coping skills for managing the often stressful process of dealing with schizophrenic family members.

Social Skills Training addresses one often-overlooked aspect of schizophrenia: the impact that schizophrenia can have on social interactions and communication. By teaching social skills, individuals can learn (or relearn) the principles of social engagement, from starting a conversation to interpreting social cues. This training can help individuals improve their ability to form and maintain meaningful relationships.

Vocational Rehabilitation and Supported Employment Programs can offer pathways for chronic schizophrenics to explore, train for, and carry out meaningful work. By forming partnerships with many employers, these programs do more than just provide job placement; they can also help schizophrenics who might otherwise be unemployed or homeless gain a sense of purpose and belonging from working in steady jobs that provide an income. For those individuals with more severe symptoms, there are also sheltered workshops that provide a safe space where they can avoid the stigma that might occur elsewhere.

Art and Music Therapy can help schizophrenics express themselves in remarkable ways, even when they cannot find the right words. By exploring their thoughts and feelings in a safe, therapeutic setting, many schizophrenics can create amazing compositions and process their inner experiences into forms that others can share with them.

Mindfulness and Meditation training can help individuals with schizophrenia explore their innermost feelings without judgment, not to mention reducing stress and promoting a sense of calm that can relieve agitation and reduce the need for tranquillizers.

Exercise also plays a crucial role in the non-drug management of schizophrenia. Regular physical activity can improve mood, reduce symptoms of anxiety and depression, and enhance overall well-being. Whether it's a walk in the park, yoga, or team sports, regular exercise can help individuals with schizophrenia reduce the risk of health problems due to prolonged inactivity. It can also help control the weight gain side effects from many medications.

While none of these non-drug therapies and interventions can be considered to be stand-alone treatments on their own, they can each play a vital role in the overall schizophrenia treatment process. Given the complex nature of schizophrenia, it's hardly surprising that a treatment approach combining multiple avenues of healing will be needed for the individuals they serve. Multiple treatment regimens also allow friends and family members to work with healthcare professionals from different disciplines to provide their loved ones with the best possible treatment.

33. Can alternative medicine help those with schizophrenia?

While alternative medicine offers a constellation of practices and remedies promising relief for many diseases, including schizophrenia, it is important to remain cautious. This is especially true for treatment approaches often lacking the empirical testing associated with more medically accepted approaches.

Alternative medicine, in the context of schizophrenia, often means combining a range of practices from the ancient to the modern, much of which depends on anecdotal evidence testifying to its effectiveness. However, navigating this diverse landscape of alternative remedies requires that people consider their use and consult with healthcare providers to ensure that such remedies don't harm more than good. Examples of alternative medication remedies that have been tried with schizophrenics include:

Omega-3 Fatty Acids: Found abundantly in fish oils, omega-3 fatty acids are a popular nutritional supplement often praised for their potential brain health benefits. Emerging research suggests that omega-3s might play a role in reducing the risk of psychosis in individuals at high risk for schizophrenia. Picture omega-3s as nurturers of the brain, offering a foundation of support for mental health, though they are not a stand-alone treatment for schizophrenia. While omega-3 fatty acid supplements can often be found in any health food store, seek medical advice to avoid potential drug interactions.

Herbal Supplements: Ginkgo biloba and other herbal supplements have long been explored for their potential benefits in improving cognitive functions among those with schizophrenia. Unfortunately, the results of these various studies tend to be inconclusive and have even shown many of these herbal supplements to have harmful interactions with conventional medications or carry their own side effects. As with omega-3 fatty acids, don't take these supplements without medical consultation.

Acupuncture: While acupuncture remains deeply embedded in traditional Chinese medicine, research on its efficacy for schizophrenia, in particular, remains limited. Despite anecdotal evidence that some schizophrenics consider it effective in role in managing symptoms like anxiety and improving overall well-being, acupuncture's value as a schizophrenia treatment remains controversial. As with other examples of alternative medication, do not consider acupuncture treatment for schizophrenics without medical advice.

These are just some examples of alternative medicine that might be considered by schizophrenics or their loved ones feeling frustrated by the lack of progress they might be experiencing. Also, people from other cultures may have greater confidence in traditional healing practices, particularly if they have used such treatments in the past. Whatever the reason for considering alternative medicine, its value of alternative medicine in treating schizophrenia cannot be dismissed completely but should never be allowed to replace conventional medicine. Those considering its use should do their own research and only in consultation with medical professionals.

34. What role do psychiatric hospitals play in helping those with schizophrenia? Can a person with schizophrenia be hospitalized against their will?

In previous eras, psychiatric hospitals gained a grim reputation which was often shrouded in mystery and misconceptions. Before the advent of antipsychotic medications and other treatments, few, if any, of those who entered these hospitals ever left again. Even today that sinister reputation still persists, though modern hospitals have evolved into crucial sanctuaries for many people grappling with schizophrenia. As are modern centers of healing, psychiatric hospitals provide comprehensive care for individuals, including acute, rehabilitative, and sometimes long-term support for those with schizophrenia.

At the core, psychiatric hospitals provide a safe haven during times of acute crisis. Schizophrenia, with its potential for severe psychotic episodes, can sometimes lead individuals into profoundly distressing states where they might pose a danger to themselves or others. As such, psychiatric hospitals allow these symptoms to be closely monitored, and the most appropriate treatments can be administered swiftly and safely. Here, the priority is to stabilize the individual, using medication adjustments, therapy, and support services to reduce the intensity of symptoms and begin the process of recovery.

Beyond immediate crisis intervention, psychiatric hospitals offer structured environments where individuals can engage with various therapeutic activities, including individual and group therapy, occupational therapy, and social skills training. These programs are designed not just to treat symptoms but to provide individuals with the skills and strategies they need to navigate life with schizophrenia. In this sense, psychiatric hospitals are not just about stabilization but about rehabilitation that prepares schizophrenics for life in the community.

In psychiatric hospitals, care is provided by a team of professionals, from psychiatrists and psychologists to nurses, social workers, and occupational therapists. This multidisciplinary approach addresses not just the medical aspects of schizophrenia but the social, emotional, and practical needs of the individual. Families and caregivers are often involved in this process, receiving education and support to create a nurturing environment both within the hospital and after discharge.

However, the question of whether people experiencing schizophrenia can be hospitalized against their will is a frightening one. In certain circumstances, yes, a person with schizophrenia can be hospitalized involuntarily. This is typically reserved for situations where the individual is unable to recognize the severity of their condition due to their symptoms and is deemed to pose a significant risk to themselves or others. Involuntary hospitalization is governed by strict legal criteria and processes, varying by jurisdiction, designed to protect the individual's rights while ensuring their safety and that of the public.

Typically, an order for involuntary hospitalization needs to be signed by a medical doctor who has conducted an assessment and determined that the person to be held is in immediate danger or poses an immediate risk to others. Such orders are only valid for a fixed period, e.g., seventy-two hours in some cases and can only be renewed by a medical panel if necessary. During this period, involuntary medication and other treatments are allowed, but medical professionals must employ their best judgment concerning patient rights.

As you can imagine, involuntary treatment raises numerous ethical and moral questions about autonomy and the right to self-determination. It's a path that needs to balance an individual's freedom with the necessity of treatment in severe cases. The decision is not taken lightly, often involving legal proceedings, medical assessments, and sometimes, court orders. The aim of such treatment is to provide necessary care while respecting the individual's rights, and, hopefully, to reach a point where such patients can continue their treatment voluntarily.

Despite the stigma still attached to psychiatric hospitals, they play a vital role in supporting many individuals with schizophrenia. This includes urgent care during crises, serving as a bridge to recovery, and offering a structured environment for rehabilitation. Though the use of involuntary hospitalization remains controversial, such involuntary treatment is aimed at balancing individual rights with basic considerations about treatment and safety. Whether or not someone with schizophrenia will need hospitalization depends on the symptoms they are displaying and how well they can function in the community with the proper treatment.

35. What types of support systems are beneficial for individuals with schizophrenia?

Providing proper support for people dealing with schizophrenia means more than just medical treatment. It also means having a reliable network of people who can be called on as needed to help schizophrenics overcome hurdles in their recovery and to guide the treatment process. Members of this support network can include:

Family and Friends: The role of friends and family in providing emotional support, understanding, and acceptance cannot be understated. Unconditional support from loved ones who are properly educated about schizophrenia can help schizophrenics: cope more effectively with whatever symptoms they are experiencing, give them the confidence to deal with their treatment and recovery, and, by watching for signs of potential relapse, help ensure timely intervention and support.

Mental Health Professionals: Psychiatrists, psychologists, and therapists are the most well-known providers of services for managing schizophrenia. They don't just offer expertise in applying medical treatment but also in providing psychotherapy, counseling, and crisis management. For this reason, mental health professionals often need to be available around the clock for when the inevitable emergencies arise, day or night. They also provide regular appointments and therapy sessions allowing them to check in on those being treated and to allow them to share their own concerns about symptoms, side effects, or the general difficulties of living in the community.

Peer Support Groups: Connecting with others who have similar experiences can be a beacon of hope and understanding for people with schizophrenia and their loved ones. Peer support groups are available not only for those with schizophrenia, but also for parents, spouses, family members, and friends who need to share their own stories. These peer support groups offer a unique space where individuals can share their stories, challenges, and victories without fear of judgment. These groups provide not just emotional support but also practical advice and insights that only facing similar challenges can offer. Not only do treatment groups help fight isolation, but they can let people in need build new support networks and strengthen existing ones.

Community Mental Health Services: These services extend the network of support into the wider community, offering access to resources such as case management, housing assistance, and vocational training. They act as bridges, connecting individuals with schizophrenia to social service agencies, potential employers, and housing facilities which help them achieve their personal goals. The support offered by community mental health services can be invaluable, particularly for those who are homeless or jobless. Unfortunately, community mental health services are most commonly found in larger cities, meaning that those living in rural areas often need to travel long distances to get services.

Online Support Platforms: In the digital age, support extends into the virtual world, providing an accessible, often anonymous, space for individuals to seek information, advice, and community. Online forums, social media groups, and mental health apps offer platforms where individuals can connect, share, and learn from others across the globe. This digital support system breaks down geographical and social barriers, offering a lifeline to those who might otherwise feel isolated.

Educational and Vocational Programs: People experiencing schizophrenia can often find their education and career goals being seriously disrupted as a result. This is why specialized programs offering educational assistance and supported employment can play a crucial role in helping schizophrenics get their lives back on track. These programs aid in skill development and job placement, boost self-esteem, and help foster a sense of purpose and independence.

As we can see here, the support systems for individuals with schizophrenia are as diverse as the needs and experiences of those they aim to assist. Each system can play its own role in providing schizophrenics with a more fulfilling and independent life. They also provide a network of support which shows that recovery is possible, that understanding is available, and that many people are willing to help.

Living with Schizophrenia

36. How does schizophrenia affect a person's daily life?

Schizophrenia is a complex, chronic mental health disorder that doesn't just impact the individual diagnosed with it, but also has a profound impact on their daily life and how they interact with others. Imagine waking up to a world where you have trouble understanding what's real and what isn't. For someone with schizophrenia, distinguishing between reality and hallucinations or delusions can be a daily struggle. These hallucinations aren't just figments of imagination; they can be as vivid and convincing as any real-life experience. The sound of a loved one calling out, the sight of a figure lurking in the corner, or the sensation of unseen hands touching you can all feel intensely real. This constant battle with hallucinations can turn routine activities like commuting, working, or simply resting at home into frightening experiences.

Delusions, another hallmark of schizophrenia, can also warp a person's ability to perceive reality. Due to such delusions, people experiencing schizophrenic symptoms might believe they are being spied on, targeted by a conspiracy, or endowed with extraordinary powers or missions. These beliefs can make them behave in ways that might seem irrational or bizarre to outsiders. As a result, trusting other people and communicating with friends, family, and co-workers become impossible as they isolate themselves from others.

Schizophrenia can also affect memory, attention, and the ability to organize thoughts. Following conversations, maintaining a train of thought, or doing complex tasks becomes harder. Imagine trying to focus on a work assignment or even a casual conversation when your thoughts are scattered, or you struggle to remember important details. It can often seem easier for someone trying to function at school or work to give up completely.

And then, there are the emotional symptoms which people with schizophrenia might exhibit. Someone showing a lack of interest in activities they once enjoyed or no emotion at all can often be misconstrued, further straining relationships. At times, they might also experience bouts of depression or anxiety, adding another layer to their daily challenges.

Naturally enough, the symptoms displayed by many often lead to social isolation, loneliness, and the deterioration of social skills. While they may still want to connect with others and keep their sense of normalcy, their ability to reach out and maintain relationships can be severely impaired.

The daily life of someone with schizophrenia also involves navigating the healthcare system, from diagnosis to treatment. This includes regular visits to healthcare providers, adhering to medication regimes that might come with challenging side effects, and participating in therapy sessions. Even with the support of loved ones and mental health professionals, the treatment needed to manage the symptoms of schizophrenia is an additional source of stress that can frequently disrupt daily life.

Despite these challenges, it's important to remember that people with schizophrenia can still have a fulfilling life with the help of loved ones, effective treatment, and a strong safety net. Still, understanding the daily impact of schizophrenia on an individual's life is crucial for fostering compassion and support. With the necessary awareness and empathy, people can learn to overcome misinformation and stigma and provide a more supportive environment for those living with schizophrenia.

37. Can people with schizophrenia live independently? What role do long-term care facilities play in helping those with schizophrenia?

Living with schizophrenia is undeniably challenging, yet it is still possible to live an independent life with the right support. Many individuals diagnosed with schizophrenia can manage their symptoms effectively, hold down productive jobs, maintain relationships, and live independently with the right treatment plan in place. But, the path to independence can vary significantly depending on how severe the symptoms are, the effectiveness of treatment, and what kind of support is available.

As we have already seen, whether someone with schizophrenia is able to live independently hinges on several crucial factors. Effective medication management is likely the most important, as it can significantly reduce the severity of symptoms such as delusions and hallucinations. Along with medication, therapy and psychosocial interventions are vital since they equip schizophrenics with strategies to manage everyday stressors, improve social skills, and recognize early signs of relapse. Regular check-ups and a strong support system of family, friends, and mental health professionals are also needed to provide encouragement and assistance in navigating the challenges of daily life.

Independence does not necessarily mean going it alone, however. For many people coping with schizophrenia, it can be vital to be part of a community providing access to the resources they need to manage their health. Long-term care facilities and community-based programs often play a crucial role for those who, temporarily or permanently, need a structured environment to thrive.

Long-term care facilities for individuals with schizophrenia or other mental health problems are designed to provide a supportive environment that promotes stability and healthy living. These facilities vary widely in the level of care and independence they offer, ranging from residential treatment centers with twenty-four-hour medical supervision to supported housing where individuals can live semi-independently with regular visits from mental health professionals.

By giving people with schizophrenia a structured routine, including regular meals, medications, and treatment programming, such routines help reduce stress and anxiety and make their symptoms more manageable. Moreover, these settings offer immediate access to psychiatric care and medication management, reducing the risk of relapse and ensuring that residents receive continuous care tailored to their evolving needs.

Long-term care facilities also play a vital educational role, offering programs that teach life skills such as budgeting, cooking, and job readiness. This education helps foster independence by giving residents the tools they need to eventually live on their own, whether that means returning to their community or just moving to housing with fewer restrictions.

These facilities also provide a social framework that can ease the loneliness and isolation that many people with schizophrenia experience. Living in a community of peers provides opportunities to build relationships, practice social skills, and support each other's progress. This sense of belonging can be as therapeutic as any other treatment program.

Still, the journey through long-term care is usually only a transitional phase as people with schizophrenia try for greater autonomy. Since the ultimate goal for most schizophrenics is to help them manage their symptoms effectively, the programming provided by these facilities is aimed at restoring confidence and helping patients move on to live as independently as possible.

However, long-term care can still be an option for some people dealing with schizophrenia. The decision to enter or utilize a long-term care facility is deeply personal and varies greatly depending on individual circumstances, symptoms, and stages of life. Even for those needing this extra care, treatment programming can be invaluable in helping to regain a sense of personal worth and in managing symptoms that might be overwhelming otherwise.

In conclusion, many individuals with schizophrenia can and do live independently, not to mention living fulfilling lives with personal achievements and meaningful relationships. For others, long-term care facilities offer the support and structure needed to manage their symptoms and work toward independence. These facilities are not just places of care; they can lead to greater autonomy by providing the tools and support needed to live with schizophrenia. As we have seen before, there is no one-size-fits-all solution for schizophrenia, and the help that is needed can be as diverse as the symptoms themselves.

38. How can families and caregivers support individuals with schizophrenia at home?

Supporting a family member with schizophrenia at home requires patience, understanding, and love. It's about fostering stability, encouraging growth, and, above all, providing unconditional support. Some of the different ways that families and caregivers can provide effective support at home include:

Understanding and Education: The first step in supporting a loved one with schizophrenia involves learning about the symptoms, treatment options, and challenges your loved one can face. We've already discussed some of the misconceptions and stigma surrounding schizophrenia, and learning to overcome them can significantly improve your ability to offer support. Improving your knowledge about schizophrenia demystifies the condition, breaks down stigma, and prepares you for the often complex care that is needed. Learning more about schizophrenia also equips you to educate others and to spread awareness and understanding within your community.

Creating a Supportive Environment: While the home environment provided is never going to be completely stress-free, reducing that stress as much as possible plays a crucial role in managing schizophrenia. Simple routines, minimal stress, and a quiet, safe space can help reduce the likelihood of episodes or relapses.

It is also essential to encourage a lifestyle that promotes mental health, such as regular sleep schedules, healthy eating habits, and physical activity. A predictable routine doesn't just help manage symptoms; it also provides a sense of security and normalcy.

Encouraging Treatment Compliance: Adhering to treatment plans, including medication and therapy, is a vital part of managing schizophrenia. Unfortunately, far too many individuals with schizophrenia may resist treatment due to worrying about side effects or even by refusing to admit that such treatment is necessary. Families can play a vital role by gently encouraging their loved ones to follow their treatment regimen, attending doctor's appointments, and actively participating in discussions with healthcare providers. Sometimes, knowing someone is there for them can make all the difference.

Developing Communication Skills: Effective communication is critical in supporting someone with schizophrenia. This involves listening actively, speaking clearly, and showing empathy and patience. It's also vital to recognize that your loved one's experiences, even if influenced by hallucinations or delusions, are very real to *them*. By validating their feelings without necessarily confirming what they are experiencing, it is possible to help maintain trust and open lines of communication.

Managing Crises: Families and caregivers should be prepared to manage crises as they occur, typically by recognizing signs of acute episodes or worsening symptoms. Having a crisis plan ready, including emergency contact numbers and a set procedure for seeking help, can provide a roadmap when someone with schizophrenia relapses. Safety for all family members, including the individual with schizophrenia, is paramount during these episodes.

Encouraging Independence and Participation: While providing support is essential, it's also important to encourage loved ones dealing with schizophrenia to be as independent as possible and to participate in daily activities. This could involve helping them set small, achievable goals, encouraging hobbies or interests, and involving them in household tasks. Even small successes can help boost self-esteem and promote a more active, engaging lifestyle.

Building a Support Network: Caring for someone with schizophrenia is not a journey you have to undertake alone. Building a network of support, including friends, extended family, healthcare providers, and community resources, can provide make the burden of care easier. Support groups, both in-person and online, can also offer valuable advice, share experiences, and provide emotional support.

Self-Care for Caregivers: Supporting a loved one with schizophrenia is profoundly rewarding but can also be emotionally and physically draining. Caregivers must remember to take care of themselves, too. This means setting aside time for personal interests, ensuring adequate rest, and seeking support when needed. Self-care is essential for maintaining emotional resilience and to prevent stress-related medical issues that can often arise.

In conclusion, supporting a friend or family member with schizophrenia at home extends beyond mere caregiving. It's about creating a nurturing environment that promotes healing, understanding, and growth. That includes education, patience, and a commitment to their well-being. While it is far too easy for many families and caregivers to "burn out" due to prolonged stress, providing this care can make a significant difference in the lives of individuals with schizophrenia, both in helping them navigate the challenges involved and to lead fulfilling lives.

39. What is the impact of schizophrenia on family members and caregivers?

There is certainly no question that the impact of schizophrenia on family members and caregivers can be profound. The extended care needed for any chronic disease, whether it be dementia or cancer, not only transforms the lives of those directly but also deeply affects their loved ones. With schizophrenia and other serious mental disorders, people providing chronic care are often marked by emotional turbulence, the need to deal with constant challenges, and helping patients navigate the often frustrating mental health treatment system. Examples of the stress that people providing chronic care experience include:

Emotional Impact: One of the most immediate effects on family members and caregivers is emotional. Watching a loved one grapple with symptoms such as hallucinations, delusions, and social withdrawal can be heart-wrenching. The person they once knew may seem to drift away, replaced by someone who is battling symptoms that others can't fully comprehend. Feelings of grief, loss, and helplessness are common as family members mourn the loss of the person they once knew and adjust to their new reality. The unpredictable nature of schizophrenia can also lead to chronic stress and anxiety among caregivers and family members. They may constantly fear the next episode or crisis, worrying about their loved one's safety and well-being. Keeping up this kind of vigilance over the long term can be emotionally and physically exhausting.

Social Impact: We have already discussed the often heartbreaking stigma that schizophrenics, and, by extension, their families, can experience. Given the misunderstandings and popular perceptions surrounding schizophrenia, friends and extended family often withdraw, unsure of how to offer support or deal with the illness. This can leave caregivers feeling lonely and unsupported, compounded by the fact that much of their time and energy is devoted to caring for their loved one, leaving little room for socializing or maintaining other relationships.

Financial and Occupational Impact: Without a doubt, the financial strain on families can be significant. Treatment for schizophrenia, including medication, therapy, and sometimes hospitalization, can be expensive, especially in countries without comprehensive healthcare coverage. Additionally, the disorder may limit the affected individual's ability to work, further straining the family's finances. Caregivers may also face their own occupational challenges. The demands of caregiving can limit their ability to work full-time or pursue career opportunities. They may have to take time off work, reduce their hours, or even quit altogether, leading to a loss of income and, in some cases, professional identity.

Physical Health Impact: The stress and demands of caregiving can have a strong effect on physical health. Chronic stress is linked to a range of health issues, including heart disease, high blood pressure, and weakened immune function. Caregivers may neglect their own health needs, skipping doctor's appointments or ignoring health problems because they are focused on their loved one's care.

Positive Impacts: While the challenges are undeniable, caring for someone with schizophrenia can also have positive impacts. Families often develop stronger bonds through their shared experiences and support for each other. Caregivers may gain a deep sense of purpose and fulfillment from their role, and many find a sense of resilience and strength they didn't know they had. This is why support and understanding are essential both for schizophrenics and their families. By educating themselves about the disorder, they can learn to find support from mental health professionals and connect with other families going through the same struggle. Caregivers also learn the importance of taking care of their own well-being and avoiding the burnout that can leave many schizophrenics isolated and even homeless.

The impact schizophrenia can have on family members and caregivers shows how important comprehensive support systems can be. Mental health services, social services, and community networks can all help, but caregivers also need to recognize the challenges involved in dealing with the often perplexing symptoms many schizophrenics experience. Still, the unyielding support of family and caregivers is a source of resilience for schizophrenics, not to mention driving home how powerful human connection can be in the face of adversity.

40. What are the implications of schizophrenia for parenting and family life?

When it comes to parenting, schizophrenia can play a profound role in stigma, stress, child welfare, and family dynamics. Understanding the impact of schizophrenia, along with providing targeted support and help, is crucial for fostering healthy family environments.

There are certainly numerous challenges for individuals with schizophrenia who are also parents. The stigma associated with mental disorders can often lead to prejudice and discrimination, particularly for children of schizophrenics, who may find themselves increasingly isolated or targets of bullying as a result. Parenting stress is another significant challenge, considering that many symptoms of schizophrenia can make daily parenting tasks and decision-making difficult, thereby increasing stress levels. As a result, such stress often worsens the symptoms of schizophrenia, creating a vicious cycle.

There is also the critical issue of child welfare involvement. Due to concerns about the ability of parents with schizophrenia to provide safe and stable environments, these families often come under the scrutiny of child welfare agencies. This can lead to increased stress and possible family separation, thus making it even harder to maintain a stable family situation.

There has been a great deal of research looking at the impact of parental schizophrenia on child development and family dynamics. Numerous studies have shown that children of schizophrenic parents are at increased risk for emotional and behavioral problems, increased risk of developing psychiatric disorders, and difficulties in academic and social settings. Coping with the needs of a schizophrenic parent can also impose considerable stress on other family members. For example, older children may take on caregiving roles prematurely. At the same time, the non-schizophrenic spouse often faces increased pressure to act as the primary caregiver for both the children and the affected partner.

However, there are effective strategies for helping parents with schizophrenia and their families. Educational programs that teach parents and children about mental illness and effective coping can help prevent worse problems from developing. Parenting skills training is another essential strategy. These programs can help individuals with schizophrenia acquire practical parenting skills, manage their emotions, and improve communication with their children. By stressing routine and structure, this training can be beneficial in creating a stable home environment.

Family therapy may also a crucial role by addressing problems with family dynamics, improving communication, and resolving family conflicts as they occur. Family therapy often provides a safe space for all family members to express their feelings and concerns, making family bonds stronger.

There are numerous examples of successful interventions and advocacy efforts aimed at supporting families affected by parental schizophrenia. Along with working with mental health professionals, there are peer support programs where parents with similar experiences share their challenges and strategies. These programs can be beneficial in providing emotional and practical support and in reducing the stigma associated with the disorder. Peer support programs can also work with advocacy groups in promoting the rights of parents with schizophrenia, ensuring they have access to necessary services, and fighting stigma and misconceptions wherever they occur.

As we can see, the implications of schizophrenia on parenting and family life are significant but having the right support structures in place can help reduce problems. Through education, tailored interventions, and robust support systems, individuals with schizophrenia can fulfill their roles as parents, and their families can thrive in supportive, understanding environments.

41. What are the impacts of schizophrenia on spirituality and religious beliefs?

Schizophrenia can have a profound impact on many aspects of a person's life, including their spirituality and religious beliefs. For many individuals dealing with schizophrenia, spirituality and religion are vital components of their identity and how they cope with the challenges posed by schizophrenia. However, the relationship that schizophrenia can have with spirituality, and religious beliefs often varies widely among individuals.

Not only do religious beliefs often provide a framework through which individuals with schizophrenia find meaning in their lives, but religious rituals can offer comfort and predictability when dealing with schizophrenic symptoms. Also, spiritual communities can offer a sense of belonging and support, which is essential for fostering resilience and promoting mental health recovery.

Many schizophrenics may choose to interpret their experiences of schizophrenia through a spiritual lens, sometimes viewing symptoms such as hallucinations or delusions as religious experiences or messages from a higher power. For some, this can reinforce their faith and spiritual practices; for others, it might lead to confusion and distress. Engagement in religious practices also varies, with some individuals finding solace in the rituals and community support. In contrast, others may feel alienated due to their symptoms or the stigma associated with mental illness.

Still, there are notable challenges in accessing spiritual support for individuals with schizophrenia. Misunderstandings about mental illness can lead to exclusion or inappropriate responses to the spiritual interpretations individuals may have of their symptoms. There have been numerous cases in which people with schizophrenia or other mental disorders were forced to undergo "exorcisms" due to the belief that their symptoms were caused by demonic possession. Additionally, the symptoms of schizophrenia, such as social withdrawal or paranoia, can make participating in community religious activities difficult. Integrating spiritual beliefs into a recovery plan is also challenging when healthcare providers may not fully understand or respect these beliefs as part of the therapeutic process.

Along with these challenges, it's also important to recognize the importance of cultural awareness in mental healthcare. Mental health professionals need to respect and understand the spiritual and religious beliefs of those with schizophrenia to provide effective support. This understanding helps develop more personalized treatment plans that consider these beliefs as being part of how individuals see themselves and how they cope with what they are experiencing. Involving spiritual leaders in mental healthcare can help ensure that all aspects of a person's well-being are addressed.

There are already prominent examples of spiritual and religious communities that are educated about mental health issues and which can act as vital support networks as a result. Some religious groups have developed specific ministries or support groups focusing on mental health and providing a safe space for individuals to explore their spirituality without judgment. You will find several examples in the Appendix.

Peer-led support groups that focus on spirituality can also play a crucial role. These groups often allow individuals to share their experiences in combining spiritual and religious lives with the challenges of living with schizophrenia. Such peer support can be incredibly validating and empowering, helping to reduce isolation and build community connections.

In conclusion, addressing the spiritual and religious needs of individuals with schizophrenia is crucial for their overall well-being and recovery. By respecting diverse beliefs, fostering inclusive communities, and incorporating collaborative care approaches, mental health professionals can better support the spiritual well-being of those affected by schizophrenia, ultimately enhancing their quality of life and resilience.

42. What's the best way to communicate with and support a friend or family member with schizophrenia?

Communicating with and supporting a friend or family member with schizophrenia requires a foundation of understanding, empathy, and patience. Forming such bonds requires both compassion and resilience, considering how schizophrenia can disrupt how people perceive, think, or feel. Finding the best way to offer support involves a blend of active listening, maintaining a positive environment, involving professional caregivers, and, most importantly, ensuring you also take care of your own well-being.

Understanding the Condition: While we have already covered the importance of educating yourself about schizophrenia, self-education is still the key to supporting someone with schizophrenia. That means learning as much as possible about symptoms such as hallucinations, delusions, and cognitive impairments. Not only does self-education promote an understanding of how to handle schizophrenia symptoms as they arise, but it can also help caregivers recognize potential signs of relapsing before it's too late. Improved knowledge can also dispel the myths surrounding schizophrenia and reduce stigma as well.

Communicating Effectively: Here are some strategies to consider when seeking to communicate with a loved one coping with schizophrenia:

- *Active Listening*: Sometimes, the best support you can offer is a willingness to hear what someone with schizophrenia is trying to say. That means listening without judgment and showing unconditional support. This can be invaluable for someone struggling to make sense of their thoughts or experiences.

- *Speaking Clearly and Simply*: Due to problems with cognitive distortions or active psychotic symptoms, schizophrenics may often have difficulty understanding what people are trying to say to them. For this reason, people trying to communicate with them need to keep their language straightforward and their messages direct to avoid misunderstandings.
- *Validating Their Feelings*: While there is not way of directly understanding or seeing what a loved one is experiencing, it's real to them. It's important to acknowledge these feelings without necessarily affirming delusional beliefs. For example, "I see that this is really upsetting you," offers validation without agreeing with a delusional perspective.

Being Patient: There are always good days and bad days, even when schizophrenics are stabilized through medication. Being patient means acknowledging that recovery and coping are ongoing processes.

Creating a Supportive Environment: A stable and supportive home environment can significantly help someone dealing with schizophrenia. While allowing for some flexibility, a set routine and structure provide a sense of safety and predictability. Encourage healthy habits like regular sleep patterns, balanced nutrition, and physical activity, which can all help manage symptoms.

Encouraging Professional Help: While support from friends and family is crucial, people with schizophrenia still need professional help, including medication, therapy, and other interventions. While many schizophrenics may be reluctant to get help, or even deny that such help is needed, it is important to make them aware that the help is there. Offer to accompany them to appointments to show support and help keep track of the information provided by healthcare professionals.

Setting Boundaries: It's important to set healthy boundaries for your well-being and to foster independence in your loved one. Be clear about what you can and cannot provide, and encourage them to engage in activities promoting independence and self-care. Boundaries help prevent caregiver burnout while ensuring the relationship remains positive and supportive.

Responding to Crisis: Be prepared for potential crises since the risk of relapse will always be there. Caregivers need to ensure that they are trained to recognize the signs of an acute episode and have a plan for how to respond, including who to call and where to go for help. Knowing these steps can reduce stress and protect your loved one and those around them during challenging times.

Support Groups and Resources: Caregivers should never overlook the value of support groups and resources, both for them and their loved ones. These can be invaluable sources of information, advice, and emotional support. Connecting with others dealing with similar challenges can provide a sense of community and understanding that is deeply comforting.

Taking Care of Yourself: While we have already discussed caregiver stress, it's important to remember that supporting someone with schizophrenia is challenging. For this reason, it is vital for caregivers to take care of their own health and well-being. Ensure enough "me time" by engaging in enjoyable activities and seeking support when needed. Remember, taking care of yourself isn't selfish; it's necessary to be able to provide support for others.

Finally, supporting a friend or family member with schizophrenia requires patience, understanding, and love. By learning more about schizophrenia, communicating effectively, creating a supportive environment, and caring for one's own well-being, caregivers can provide meaningful support that makes a significant difference in a schizophrenic's life. Through empathy and resilience, it's possible to navigate the complexities of schizophrenia together, fostering a relationship that is both supportive and enriching.

43. Are people with schizophrenia at an increased risk of being unhoused or in prison?

The intersection of schizophrenia, homelessness, and involvement in the criminal justice system is a complex issue. Due to failures in the system, stigma surrounding mental illness, and gaps in mental healthcare, people with schizophrenia face numerous challenges that can, unfortunately, increase their vulnerability to homelessness and imprisonment. As to why this can happen, we need to delve into how societies support those with severe mental health conditions and where the social net often falls short.

Vulnerability to Homelessness: People with schizophrenia are at a heightened risk of homelessness for numerous reasons. The symptoms of schizophrenia, such as difficulty maintaining concentration, erratic behavior, and social withdrawal, can make holding down a job or maintaining support networks extremely difficult.

Without employment, financial resources dwindle, making it difficult to afford housing. As well, the social isolation that often accompanies schizophrenia can lead to a lack of family or community support. When individuals with schizophrenia lose touch with their support networks, they have fewer resources to rely on during crises, making homelessness a looming threat. Additionally, the cognitive aspects of the disorder can make managing daily tasks, such as paying rent on time or maintaining a rental agreement, more challenging. This problem is often worsened by the scarcity of affordable housing and the inadequacy of social safety nets in many regions. When individuals with schizophrenia seek help, they may find that resources are stretched thin, with long waiting lists for subsidized housing or insufficient emergency shelter beds. This gap between the need for supportive housing and its availability is a major factor in the homelessness risk for people with schizophrenia.

Increased Risk of Imprisonment: There are also major challenges when schizophrenics come in contact with the criminal justice system. Encounters with law enforcement can escalate if officers are not trained to recognize and appropriately respond to mental health crises. Misunderstandings and the unpredictable behavior associated with schizophrenia can lead to arrests for minor offenses or situations that would have been better managed by mental health professionals. Once in the criminal justice system, people with schizophrenia may not receive the care they need. The symptoms of their condition can make navigating the legal system more difficult, from communicating with lawyers to understanding the proceedings. The lack of adequate mental healthcare within prisons and jails further complicates their ability to cope with the environment and potentially make their condition worse. This is especially true if schizophrenics refuse to take their medication out of the belief that they are not mentally ill or a fear that they might be "muscled" for their medication by other inmates.

Addressing the risks of homelessness and imprisonment for individuals with schizophrenia requires a multifaceted approach. Increased investment in mental healthcare, including early intervention programs, comprehensive treatment options, and ongoing support, is critical. Such support not only helps people manage the symptoms of schizophrenia but also assists individuals in maintaining employment and housing.

Supportive housing programs that offer a stable living environment coupled with access to mental health services can significantly reduce the risk of homelessness. These programs recognize the importance of addressing mental health needs as part of the solution to housing insecurity. Unfortunately, such programs often have long waiting lists, which can make the problem substantially worse.

Training for law enforcement and other first responders in mental health crisis intervention can help prevent unnecessary incarcerations. These programs equip officers with the skills to de-escalate situations and direct individuals toward the help they need rather than into the criminal justice system.

Community-based mental health services that include assertive outreach teams can engage individuals with schizophrenia who are at risk of homelessness or involvement with the criminal justice system. By providing consistent and proactive support, these teams can ensure that individuals receive the care they need to manage their symptoms and navigate daily challenges.

In summary, while individuals with schizophrenia face an increased risk of homelessness and imprisonment, these outcomes are not inevitable. By prioritizing mental healthcare, supportive housing, specialized training for first responders, and community-based services, it can be possible to reduce these risks. It's a matter of viewing individuals with schizophrenia not as statistics but as members of the community deserving of empathy, support, and the opportunity to lead fulfilling lives.

44. How have media portrayals of schizophrenia impacted popular perceptions of the condition?

How popular media portrays schizophrenia has significantly shaped public perceptions of mental illness, often in ways that distort and simplify the complex realities of living with schizophrenia. The influence of movies, television shows, news reports, and online content on societal attitudes cannot be understated. How schizophrenia can be presented deeply impacts the way people with schizophrenia are viewed, treated, and understood in everyday life.

One of the most notable impacts of media portrayals is the reinforcement of stereotypes and stigma. Films and television shows have historically depicted individuals with schizophrenia as dangerous or violent, something that contributes to the kind of stigma that makes it harder for them to seek help or achieve acceptance. The misconception that schizophrenia leads to violence has been debunked by research showing that individuals with mental health conditions are more likely to be victims rather than perpetrators of violence.

The popular media also tends to dramatize or inaccurately represent the symptoms of schizophrenia. Hallucinations, particularly auditory ones, are frequently depicted, while other important aspects of the condition, such as negative symptoms (e.g., apathy, lack of emotion, and poor social functioning), receive less attention. This selective representation can lead to unrealistic expectations and perceptions about the challenges faced by those with schizophrenia.

For many people, television, movies, and online content are their primary sources of information about mental health conditions. When these portrayals are misleading or sensationalized, they can lead to misconceptions that affect how individuals with schizophrenia are perceived and treated in society. For example, if schizophrenics are continually shown as violent or unpredictable, the public may be unnecessarily fearful or suspicious of individuals with the condition, impacting social integration and support.

But it's not just the popular media that can reinforce misconceptions about schizophrenia; the news media can play a role as well, often by focusing on extreme cases or incidents involving violence. This skewed reporting can reinforce the false association between schizophrenia and dangerous behavior while overshadowing the stories of those with schizophrenia who lead stable, peaceful lives. Furthermore, the news media focuses on crises rather than recovery or success stories, exploring the potential for positive outcomes with proper support and treatment.

Unfortunately, how schizophrenia is portrayed in the media can also affect individuals diagnosed with the condition. Negative stereotypes about schizophrenia and other serious mental illnesses can shape how those affected might see themselves. Not only can it lead to decreased self-esteem or self-stigma, but it also makes them more reluctant to disclose their diagnosis or seek help. The stigma against mental illness can be especially strong in many traditional cultures, with schizophrenics facing family pressure to keep their condition hidden and not to ask for treatment.

In recent years, advocacy groups have called for more responsible and accurate portrayals of schizophrenia and mental health conditions in general. Rather than focusing on sensational news stories and the popular media, media portrayals of schizophrenia are beginning to reflect the many challenges, triumphs, and daily living they experience. Breaking down the old stereotypes makes it possible to promote understanding and highlight the importance of support and compassion. As awareness grows, future portrayals will hopefully become more accurate in showing the realities of living with schizophrenia.

45. What are the impacts of schizophrenia on cultural identity and heritage?

Schizophrenia profoundly impacts individuals across all aspects of their lives, including their cultural identity and heritage. Cultural identity plays a significant role in how individuals perceive their symptoms, seek help, and cope with their condition. The relationship between schizophrenia and cultural identity is multifaceted, reflecting broader societal attitudes toward mental health, individual and communal beliefs, and the diversity of coping mechanisms grounded in cultural heritage.

Cultural identity and heritage significantly influence the experiences of individuals with schizophrenia. These elements not only affect how symptoms are understood and expressed but also how they are received by the community. In some cultures, symptoms of schizophrenia might be interpreted through spiritual or supernatural frameworks, which can affect both the stigma associated with the illness and the support the individual receives. For example, in some communities, hallucinations or unusual behavior may be seen as spiritual visitations or demonic possession rather than symptoms of a psychiatric condition, affecting both acceptance and ostracization within the community. Incidents in which people with schizophrenia are forced to undergo exorcisms are hardly uncommon.

Research shows a wide diversity in how different cultures perceive mental illness, approach help-seeking behavior, and express preferences for types of treatments. Cultural beliefs can significantly influence whether individuals with schizophrenia seek help from medical professionals, traditional healers, or a combination of both. Treatment preferences can also vary; for instance, some might prefer medication, others psychotherapy, and some might lean toward herbal medicines or spiritual counselling, depending on their cultural background.

People with schizophrenia often face significant challenges in navigating these cultural norms while seeking and receiving care. The stigma of mental illness can also vary greatly between cultures but generally leads to marginalization and decreased social support. Families in some cultures even go so far as to keep their schizophrenic family members hidden in basements or attics to avoid the shame of having someone in their family with mental illness.

Even when seeking out mental healthcare, many healthcare systems often do not adequately meet the cultural needs and beliefs of diverse populations. This can frequently hinder effective treatment and recovery. Acknowledging the complex cultural needs of patients and their families remains a challenging task that requires sensitivity and adaptability from healthcare providers.

In recent years, healthcare providers have developed more culturally sensitive assessments to ensure that the treatment process remains respectful and relevant to the patient's cultural background. Collaborative care planning involving patients, their families, and even traditional healers can help develop treatments that respect cultural identities while effectively managing the illness.

And there are certainly examples which highlight the benefits of culturally tailored treatment. For instance, community-based programs incorporating elements of specific cultural practices, such as community gatherings, traditional storytelling, or spiritual rituals, can help make treatment settings more inclusive and supportive. Peer support networks, including people from the patient's culture, can offer their own shared experiences, thus reducing feelings of isolation.

Furthermore, partnerships between healthcare providers and community leaders or cultural figures can provide a deeper understanding and integration of cultural practices into care plans. These partnerships can also help educate communities about schizophrenia and combat the kind of stigma that might make community members unwilling to seek help in the first place.

As we have seen, dealing with schizophrenia requires a comprehensive, culturally informed treatment approach that respects and integrates individuals' cultural backgrounds. By embracing cultural diversity and acknowledging its significance in treatment and recovery, healthcare providers can support the well-being of individuals with schizophrenia, making their treatment more effective and respectful of cultural heritage.

46. What efforts are being made to raise awareness about and destigmatize schizophrenia?

We've already covered how negative media portrayals can reinforce misconceptions about schizophrenia and undermine the recovery process. However, mental health advocates are working to change this with new initiatives to overcome such misconceptions and promote greater understanding. Examples include:

Educational Campaigns: One of the primary strategies to destigmatize schizophrenia involves education. Numerous organizations worldwide, including the National Alliance on Mental Illness (NAMI) in the United States and Mind in the UK, have launched educational campaigns that aim to dispel myths and provide accurate information about schizophrenia. These campaigns often target schools, workplaces, and communities, offering workshops, informational materials, and presentations that cover the nature of schizophrenia, its symptoms, treatment options, and the realities of living with the condition. These campaigns hope to reduce fear and misunderstanding by replacing misinformation with facts.

Social Media and Digital Platforms: As the world grows more digital, social media and online platforms have become powerful tools for raising awareness and challenging stigma. Advocacy groups, individuals with lived experience, and mental health professionals utilize blogs, podcasts, videos, and social media campaigns to share stories, disseminate research findings, and offer support. Hashtags and social media movements help amplify voices that might otherwise go unheard, creating spaces for dialogue and community building.

Peer Support and Life Experience Sharing: Sharing personal stories of living with schizophrenia can play a profound role in humanizing the disorder and breaking down stigma. Peer support groups, either online or in person, provide safe spaces for individuals to share their experiences, challenges, and successes. These narratives can shift perceptions, showing the person behind the diagnosis and the possibility of a fulfilling life despite the challenges. Furthermore, public speaking engagements and media appearances by individuals with schizophrenia help to counteract stereotypes and showcase resilience.

Advocating Legislation: While mental health organizations and advocacy groups have been lobbying for better legislation to help the mentally ill, this has proven to be an uphill battle in many places. By stressing that mental health is as important as physical health, advocacy groups have had some success in increasing funding for mental health education, research, and providing better access to mental health services. Much more needs to be done, however.

Training for Healthcare Providers and Law Enforcement: Training programs for healthcare providers and law enforcement personnel are essential in promoting better care for people with schizophrenia and other serious mental illness. These programs need to focus on improving understanding of mental health conditions, teaching skills for compassionate interaction, and promoting *de-escalation* techniques in crisis situations. Better informed and empathetic responses from professionals can significantly reduce negative encounters and reinforce a more supportive approach to individuals experiencing symptoms of schizophrenia.

International Education Campaigns: International observances such as World Mental Health Day provide an opportunity to spotlight schizophrenia alongside broader mental health issues. And they are especially important in countries which lack proper resources to help people in need. Using public events, media campaigns, and educational community activities, advocacy groups are raising awareness about schizophrenia and other mental health disorders along with promoting dialogue about what can be done about it in diverse communities worldwide.

Increasing Research into Mental Illness: Ongoing research into schizophrenia is intended to increase understanding and treatment and to help guide public discourse. Academic institutions and researchers play a critical role in demystifying schizophrenia, with their findings providing a solid basis for educational materials and advocacy efforts. By highlighting the biological, psychological, and social aspects of schizophrenia, research challenges simplistic notions and fosters a more nuanced understanding.

As these different initiatives continue to gain momentum, there is hope for a future where schizophrenia can be understood without prejudice or misconceptions. Ultimately, allowing people affected by schizophrenia to lead regular lives free of stigma and fear can only benefit us all as a society.

47. What are the impacts of schizophrenia on aging and geriatric care?

As individuals with schizophrenia grow older, the impact that their condition can have on geriatric care becomes far more challenging. Older adults with schizophrenia often face unique issues that require careful attention to promote healthy aging and improve their quality of life. Such challenges include cognitive decline, physical health issues, and social isolation—all of which can complicate care and significantly affect their quality of life.

One of the primary challenges in aging with schizophrenia is cognitive decline. While this is a problem faced by all seniors over time, such a mental decline is often worse for those with schizophrenia compared to seniors without serious mental health issues. Since the long-term effects of schizophrenia and its treatments can profoundly affect brain functioning over time, the cognitive challenges that can result often make daily living and self-care increasingly difficult, impacting medication management and the ability to comply with treatment.

Physical health problems are also more prevalent in older adults with schizophrenia. Conditions such as cardiovascular disease, diabetes, and respiratory diseases occur at higher rates in this population, partly due to lifestyle factors such as low physical activity, poor diet, and high rates of smoking. All of these factor complicate the management of schizophrenia and increase the risk of mortality.

Social isolation is another significant concern. Older adults with schizophrenia may have spent a lifetime coping with the stigma associated with mental illness, which can lead to withdrawal from social interactions and community engagement. This isolation can worsen symptoms and lead to further cognitive and physical health decline.

There are also the problems that older adults with schizophrenia often face in accessing high-quality care. Available evidence indicates that these individuals receive less medical care for physical health problems compared to those without mental health disorders. The quality of care can also be compromised by a healthcare system that is not always equipped to address the complex needs of aging psychiatric patients. Outcomes for these individuals tend to be poorer, with higher hospitalization rates, longer hospital stays, and more significant health-related expenses.

Given the increased geriatric needs of individuals with schizophrenia, they must follow the lifestyle factors associated with healthy aging. These include proactive management of related physical illnesses, regular cognitive and physical assessments, and interventions to increase social support and community engagement. Other lifestyle interventions, such as promoting physical activity, nutritional support, and smoking cessation programs, can also be extremely effective.

Innovative models of care have been developed in recent years to help seniors with schizophrenia stay healthy. Community-based services are increasingly being used to provide comprehensive outpatient care, including mobile health teams and day-treatment programs that offer both social and medical services. Supportive housing options also play a critical role by providing stable housing, on-site care, and support services. Not only do such services address the psychiatric and physical health needs of geriatric patients, but they can also improve community and social interactions.

Examples of successful treatment programming for aging mental health patients include specialized geriatric psychiatry services, which focus on the unique needs of older adults by combining expertise in aging and mental health. Another example is the use of technology, such as telepsychiatry, to improve access to psychiatric care and support for older adults living in remote or underserved areas.

Overall, addressing the challenges faced by older adults with schizophrenia requires a comprehensive, integrated approach that considers the interplay of mental health, physical health, cognitive function, and social well-being. By focusing on person-centered care and interdisciplinary collaboration and by implementing innovative care models, it is possible to significantly improve the quality of life and outcomes for this vulnerable population.

48. What are the impacts of schizophrenia on end-of-life and palliative care?

While schizophrenia can affect health treatment throughout an individual's life, this can also extend to the realm of end-of-life care. As people continue to age, the need for palliative care is becoming more critical and providing such care for people with schizophrenia is a major challenge. Not only are chronic schizophrenics requiring end-of-life and palliative care services forced to deal with a healthcare system that can accommodate people with significant mental health problems, but many palliative care workers lack the necessary training to handle the special needs of long-term schizophrenics.

One of the primary challenges for individuals with schizophrenia nearing the end of life is the pervasive stigma associated with the condition. This stigma can influence the attitudes of healthcare providers and result in suboptimal care. Additionally, communication barriers can arise due to difficulties expressing thoughts and emotions or understanding complex medical information. These barriers make it harder for patients to report their needs and preferences for end-of-life care.

Sadly, the healthcare system itself often presents obstacles. The care for individuals with schizophrenia can be highly fragmented, with inadequate coordination between mental health services and other medical care providers. This fragmentation can lead to inconsistencies in care and difficulties in comprehensively addressing the needs of patients at the end of life.

Evidence to date suggests significant differences in how individuals with schizophrenia use palliative care compared to the general population. These individuals are less likely to engage in advance care planning or to have documented end-of-life care preferences. Unless they have family members to make these decisions for them, palliative care patients with schizophrenia often have to deal with crisis-driven care that might ignore their actual wishes and deny them the chance to die with dignity.

To address these issues, it is crucial to promote advanced care planning among individuals with schizophrenia. This involves encouraging discussions about end-of-life care preferences early in the course of treatment and revisiting these preferences as circumstances change. Respecting autonomy is central to this process, ensuring that patients are actively involved in decisions about their care, to the extent that their condition allows.

Palliative care patients with schizophrenia also need emotional support, including helping them restore their contact with family members who might help them overcome the isolation that many individuals with schizophrenia experience, especially as they approach the end of life. For this reason, individuals with schizophrenia who require palliative care often require care workers with the mental health expertise to manage psychiatric symptoms alongside medical treatment for other co-morbid conditions.

When providing end-of-life care to individuals with schizophrenia, is essential that this care prioritize the patient's own values and preferences and adapt interventions to meet their specific needs. Compassionate communication is also crucial, involving clear, respectful, and empathetic dialogue that acknowledges the dignity of the patient. Given the frequent stigma that people with schizophrenia face, especially when facing the end of life, reminding them of their inherent value and worth is also an important part of palliative care.

Several examples highlight effective end-of-life care practices for individuals with schizophrenia. Specialized training programs for palliative care providers that focus on the unique needs of psychiatric patients can improve care delivery. Collaborative care models that include mental health professionals, palliative care specialists, and primary care providers can ensure comprehensive management of both psychiatric and physical health needs.

In summary, enhancing end-of-life and palliative care for individuals with schizophrenia requires targeted efforts to overcome stigma, promote patient-centered planning, and make palliative care practices more humane. By focusing on these areas, healthcare providers can significantly improve the quality of life and dignity of individuals with schizophrenia in their final stages.

49. What are the long-term impacts of schizophrenia on society and public health?

Because schizophrenia is a chronic mental health disorder that can require lifetime care, treating the millions of people affected worldwide imposes a significant socioeconomic burden on public health and society. Healthcare costs associated with schizophrenia are already astronomical and will only rise in future. These costs include expenses for acute care, long-term treatment, and psychiatric services. Individuals with schizophrenia often require a range of services from hospitalization to ongoing outpatient care, which can be costly. Furthermore, productivity loss is a major issue, as the onset of schizophrenia typically occurs in young adulthood, affecting individuals' ability to complete education and maintain steady employment. For that matter, family members caring for schizophrenic loved ones can also face productivity loss due to time lost from work. Social welfare expenditures are also higher for this group, as individuals often require government assistance for basic living and medical expenses due to their reduced capacity to work.

Research into health trends has shown enormous disparities in life expectancy, with individuals with schizophrenia living on average 15–20 years less than the general population. This reduced life expectancy is due to a combination of factors, including increased prevalence of physical health conditions such as cardiovascular disease, higher rates of suicide, and lifestyle factors like smoking and poor diet. The quality of life for individuals with schizophrenia can also be significantly impaired due to disrupted social relationships, reduced functional ability, and the impact of stigma and discrimination. Moreover, social determinants of health, such as access to quality healthcare, safe housing, and supportive social networks, can also be affected by creating a cycle of vulnerability and marginalization.

To reduce the societal burden of schizophrenia, it is vital to diagnose and treat the symptoms of schizophrenia as early as possible. Not only can early intervention programs be used to treat schizophrenia as soon as symptoms appear, but they can also improve long-term outcomes by delaying or preventing later problems and improving the overall quality of life for those affected. Examples of early intervention programs include integrated care models, which combine psychiatric care with other health services, improve their overall health status, and reduce hospitalizations and healthcare costs. Community-based support services can also be effective in providing ongoing rehabilitation, housing support, and employment assistance, helping individuals with schizophrenia integrate into society and lead more fulfilling lives.

Investing in mental health promotion and prevention efforts is clearly needed to offset the long-term impacts of schizophrenia on society. This means improving access to mental healthcare, improving the quality of care, and investing in better programs for education, housing, and food security. Not only can this substantially improve the lives of individuals with schizophrenia, but it can help prevent mental health problems for everyone. Public awareness campaigns and education in schools and workplaces can also play a significant role in reducing the stigma and discrimination associated with mental health conditions.

Accomplishing all of this means improving advocacy, creating better legislation, and promoting more public-private partnerships to ensure mental health equity and social justice for individuals with schizophrenia. Advocacy groups are major in influencing public policies and ensuring that mental health remains a priority. Policy reforms can help improve access to health services, secure funding for research and support services, and protect the rights of individuals with mental health. Furthermore, public-private partnerships can help bring it all together through improved mental healthcare delivery and support, better resources and expertise, and forming support networks to enhance care accessibility and quality.

Unfortunately, schizophrenia will continue to have significant long-term impacts on public health and society, not to mention profound socioeconomic burdens on healthcare systems around the world. The only way to mitigate these impacts and improve the lives of individuals affected by schizophrenia is through early intervention, integrated care, and community support, and by investing in broader public health initiatives and advocating for policy reforms.

Case Studies

Case 1. Anna's Triumph over Early-Onset Schizophrenia

Anna's life took an unexpected turn during her freshman year at college. While she expected to face challenges as she got used to living away from home and immersing herself in the college experience, she found herself grappling with perplexing and frightening symptoms. Along with the persistent belief that she was being constantly watched, she became aware of whispering voices only she could hear. As these symptoms intensified, Anna's ability to concentrate on her studies waned, and her social life began to crumble as she became more isolated from her fellow students and friends. She found herself withdrawing more and more as she became trapped in a world that seemed increasingly unreal and hostile.

The transition to college life is challenging for most young adults, but for Anna, these bewildering symptoms were terrifying. At first, she attributed what she was experiencing to the stress and sleepless nights caused by typical college pressure. However, as her condition worsened, it became clear that what she was experiencing was far from ordinary. Realizing that she might be dealing with something serious came after a particularly alarming episode when the voices she was hearing started urging her to get away from the "bad people" who lived in her dormitory.

Concerned by her deteriorating state, Anna finally admitted what was happening to her parents, who immediately encouraged her to seek professional help. Fortunately, her college had a counseling center, and after opening up to one of the counsellors, she was sent to a local psychiatrist. A thorough psychiatric evaluation followed, including medical and psychological testing. In a meeting with the psychiatrist afterward, Anna, along with her parents, was told that she was in the early stages of schizophrenia. This moment was pivotal—it was both a shock and a relief. While the diagnosis gave what she was experiencing a name and a direction for treatment, it also meant that her life would be forever changed. Along with the fear of living with a chronic mental health condition, she was also typical of most people her age in not understanding what schizophrenia was and whether the diagnosis meant that she was "crazy."

Determined to deal with this new diagnosis, Anna and her parents worked to educate themselves about schizophrenia and what it meant for her future. Based on what they learned and in consultation with the doctor, Anna began a comprehensive treatment regimen that included antipsychotic medication to control her symptoms and supportive counselling to help her cope with the emotional and psychological aspects of schizophrenia. The medication helped quiet the voices and curbed the delusions, allowing her to regain a sense of control. The therapy began with individual sessions to provide a safe space to express her fears and frustrations and to learn strategies for managing her condition. Then, when Anna was deemed to be ready, she was placed in a therapy group with others going through symptoms similar to hers. By sharing her story with fellow patients and learning what they had experienced as well, Anna learned better ways of coping with her symptoms.

Gradually, as her symptoms became manageable, Anna felt confident enough to return to her classes, albeit part-time. While she was reluctant to face her fellow students at first, they welcomed her enthusiastically and had nothing but praise for how she was coping. She also started volunteering at a local community center, a turning point in her recovery. Volunteering not only helped her rebuild her self-esteem but also reconnected her with the community, easing the loneliness that had so deeply affected her.

Over the next several years, Anna's resilience and the support from her healthcare team, family, and new friends she made through volunteering helped her navigate her condition. Her life took on a new rhythm, marked by small victories and occasional setbacks. However, she met each challenge with the help of her support network, including her therapists, fellow volunteers, and college friends who admired her courage and determination.

Anna's journey from isolation to a connected and hopeful existence showed how effective early intervention and personalized care can be in managing schizophrenia. Not only did she return to school full-time and complete her degree, but she also became an advocate for mental health awareness, using her story to inspire others facing similar battles. Anna's journey illustrates the critical importance of recognizing mental health symptoms early, seeking appropriate care, and getting the necessary community support. By sharing her story, Anna hopes to reduce the stigma associated with schizophrenia and encourage others to seek help without fear of judgment.

Analysis

Anna's experience with schizophrenia during her first year of college highlights several key points in the management of mental health disorders, particularly the importance of early detection and intervention. Initially, she faced significant challenges, including auditory hallucinations and delusions that led to social isolation and academic difficulties. While Anna initially dismissed these symptoms as being caused by mere stress from college life, telling her parents about them proved to be the turning point since they recognized that these symptoms couldn't be ignored.

After her parents urged her to seek professional help, the psychiatric examination she underwent led to her being diagnosed as being in the early stages of schizophrenia. Once this diagnosis was made, she was promptly treated with psychotropic medications and individual therapy to help manage her symptoms. Though finding the right balance between medication therapy and counseling can take time, Anna's treatment soon allowed her to regain control over her life, including being able to return to college, albeit part-time.

Furthermore, Anna's case illustrates the importance of a supportive environment in the recovery process. By volunteering and engaging with her community, she not only rebuilt her social life but also regained her self-esteem and confidence, which had been eroded by her illness. The support she gained from her family, healthcare providers, and new social connections played a critical role in her recovery.

Overall, Anna's journey underscores the effectiveness of comprehensive care in managing schizophrenia, involving both medical treatment and social rehabilitation. Her story demonstrates that it is possible to lead a fulfilling life despite the challenges of living with a mental health disorder.

Case 2. John's Unmanaged Schizophrenia Leads to Homelessness

John's symptoms began subtly during his mid-twenties, though he dismissed the occasional whispers and shadows at the edge of his vision as being due to stress or lack of sleep. As time passed, however, the whispers grew into voices and the shadows into strange visions which were often terrifying. He also began experiencing severe delusions and disorganized thoughts that threw his life into a downward spiral.

While John was a skilled carpenter known for his fine craftsmanship, his deteriorating mental state began affecting his professional life. His employers eventually let him go, citing performance issues and decreased reliability. Without a steady income, John struggled to keep up with rent, and his social life dwindled due to his erratic behavior and strange beliefs brought on by his untreated condition. Within a year, John found himself living on the streets, which only deepened his isolation and worsened. Without any of the critical support systems most of us take for granted, John's life became increasingly desperate.

Ironically, the turning point in his life came when John was caught shoplifting in a small grocery store. Instead of pressing charges, the store owner, noticing John's odd behavior and disjointed speech, called for medical help. Rather than being arrested, as he probably expected, John was sent to a psychiatric hospital for an assessment instead. While he was angry at first, dealing with mental health professionals for the first time in his life was a revelation for him. Not only were they not put off by his odd behavior, but he could finally open up about symptoms he was afraid to share with anyone. Finally, after a psychiatric assessment to rule out other possible explanations for his symptoms, John was formally diagnosed with schizophrenia. While he was apprehensive at first about being labeled as mentally ill, especially considering he had been afraid of being thought "crazy" for so long, this diagnosis meant that real treatment could finally begin.

John soon found that being placed on antipsychotic medication helped mute many of the symptoms that had frightened him for so long. He was also provided with housing in a community care facility where he received regular counseling and support. The structured environment and continued therapy gradually helped him regain some normalcy in his life, along with the tools to manage his illness.

Recovery and reintegration into society were slow but steady. As John's condition stabilized, he began to engage with the community around him. After starting with individual counseling, he soon graduated to group therapy, which allowed him to interact with others who shared many of the same experiences he had. He even started volunteering at the very store he had once tried to shoplift from. Not only did this help to rebuild his self-esteem, but it also demonstrated that he could be trusted once more.

John's story didn't end with him regaining his old life but rather starting a new chapter where he could use his experience to advocate for mental health awareness and help others get off the street. He is busy speaking at community centers and writing about his experiences. Through his advocacy, he demonstrates the need for accessible mental health services and the importance of community support systems. By helping to change how society views and treats mental illnesses, John hopes to save others from enduring the loneliness and despair of being homeless and mentally ill.

While John's story is hardly unique, given the many homeless mentally ill in cities across the world, helping them escape the streets and getting the necessary treatment remains an enormous challenge. Many homeless, mentally ill people like John may find themselves drifting into the prison system or becoming targets for abuse. Being on the stress also means a drastically shortened life span since they are often cut off from medical and social services that they might need. Being homeless can also leave them prone to dying or exposure or malnutrition since they often fall between the cracks of social safety nets aimed at protecting them. Helping the homeless and mentally ill underscores a critical lesson: the profound impact of accessible mental health services and the transformative power of community compassion and support. John's life, once marked by confusion and loss, now brings hope and understanding to others, showing that with the right support, recovery is not just possible but can be a gateway to a new purposeful life.

Analysis

John's decade-long struggle with undiagnosed schizophrenia illustrates the often-heartbreaking consequences of untreated mental health issues and why support systems are so necessary. While John's symptoms were subtle and easy to ignore at first, they gradually escalated into severe delusions and disorganized thinking that made it impossible to continue with his normal life. This meant being unable to work as he could before, leading to the loss of his job and, eventually, his home. Cases like John's underscore the importance of early diagnosis and intervention in mental healthcare, which could not only have prevented his symptoms from getting worse but helping him avoid the later upheaval in his life.

The turning point in John's life came only after he was apprehended for shoplifting, which could have easily led to his being sent to prison. Instead, the compassionate response of the store owner, who recognized John's need for medical help rather than punishment, led to his eventual diagnosis and treatment. This highlights how easily community actions can alter the course of an individual's life.

John's recovery, supported by medication, counseling, and community care, shows how the homeless mentally ill can benefit from integrated treatment approaches and stable support networks. His journey from isolation to advocacy reflects not only the challenges faced by people with mental health issues but also their potential to overcome and contribute positively to society. While John's story is a positive one, there are far too many others who are not as lucky. The continuing presence of homeless mentally ill individuals in prisons, hospitals, or homeless shelters shows how vital it is to improve access to mental health services and support programs to help them reintegrate into society.

Case 3. Michael's Life in Long-Term Care

Michael was twenty-eight years old when life as he knew it began to unravel.

The early symptoms of schizophrenia, subtle yet disturbing, emerged without a clear warning. Though it is often easy to dismiss many early symptoms as signs that someone is "working too hard," the auditory hallucinations and paranoid delusions that Michael began experiencing were much harder to ignore. While he tried to hide what was happening, his coworkers and friends quickly realized that something was seriously wrong with Michael.

After a particularly alarming episode at work where Michael became disoriented and verbally abusive, his employer demanded that he seek medical help to be allowed to stay at his job. Though he wanted to argue that there was nothing wrong with him, the people in his life, including friends and family, admitted that they had been worried about him for some time. As a result, he attended the emergency department at a local hospital to ask that a psychiatrist examine him. After being assessed for several days as an inpatient medical help, Michael was formally diagnosed as being schizophrenic. This diagnosis came with mixed feelings for him and his family. While being relieved at having an explanation for his symptoms, there was also considerable fear over what this meant for his future.

Given the severity of his symptoms, which showed little improvement despite his taking medication, Michael and his family decided that a group home, offering constant care and a structured environment, would be best for him.

This environment provided regular routines and easy access to mental health professionals, which were crucial for managing his condition.

Granted, Michael wasn't happy about being placed in a group home, especially since there was no way to tell how long he would remain there. Although he had already burned his bridges when it came to holding down a full-time job or living on his own, he had no wish to lose his independence completely. While the group home staff assured him that the goal of the program was to prepare residents for life in the community but that his condition needed to be stabilized to avoid problems such as those he faced before.

Once he was living in the group home, Michael found that his life was becoming more stable. The group home's controlled setting and the treatment he received helped to control his symptoms. Medications were administered regularly, and therapy sessions were a consistent part of his schedule. However, despite these stabilizing factors, Michael struggled with social interactions. Though he still tried to connect with others, both with the group home and with visiting friends and family, his symptoms created a barrier that was difficult to overcome.

The staff at the group home worked to support Michael, not just medically but also socially. They introduced programs aimed at enhancing social skills, providing residents with tools to communicate and build relationships more effectively. For Michael, these sessions were challenging but ultimately rewarding. Slowly, he began to engage more with others, participating in group activities and occasionally sharing meals with fellow residents.

While Michael would remain in the group home setting for many years, his progress was slow but noticeable. He learned to manage his symptoms better and started to enjoy activities that had once caused him considerable anxiety. The group home environment was critical in this transformation, offering him a safe space to navigate his condition and rebuild his life within a supportive community.

Of course, there were setbacks when Michael felt overwhelmed by his slow pace of recovery and the persistent challenges in social settings. Yet, each setback was met with renewed support from the group home staff, encouraging him to keep pushing forward. As time passed, Michael found new ways to contribute to the community within the home. He took on small responsibilities, helping to organize community events and activities, which gave him a sense of purpose and belonging. These roles, though minor, were a significant step forward in his recovery, allowing him to feel valued and productive.

Today, Michael continues to live in the group home, and while challenges remain, he has formed friendships within the community which provide him with much-needed emotional support. He is also doing schoolwork to follow his own interests and remains open to the possibility of living in the community once he and his support staff feel he is ready.

Michael's story is a testament to the critical role that structured environments like group homes can play in managing schizophrenia. Stories like this also demonstrate the need for continuous, comprehensive care that addresses not only the medical but also the social needs of those living with mental health disorders. Michael's journey highlights the importance of patience, persistence, and the profound impact of a supportive community in overcoming the challenges posed by such a complex condition.

Analysis

Michael's journey with schizophrenia began in his late twenties, leading to a life now spent in a group home designed to support individuals with similar conditions. Diagnosed at a relatively young age, Michael has benefited from the structured and consistent care provided by the long-term care facility where he lives. This case study highlights the essential role such environments can play in stabilizing individuals with schizophrenia, offering regular routines, medication management, and access to mental health professionals.

The group home environment has been instrumental in reducing the severity of Michael's symptoms, allowing him to achieve a level of stability that might not have been possible otherwise. While he hopes to regain his independence and return to full-time work, he recognizes that there are many challenges which need to be overcome first. This includes his difficulties with social interactions, a common challenge for many living with schizophrenia.

Michael's situation underscores the necessity of tailored support within long-term care facilities that can adapt to the varying needs of residents, particularly those with severe mental health diagnoses. It also highlights the ongoing challenges that exist even in controlled environments, such as the need for programs that specifically address social skills and interpersonal functioning.

Overall, Michael's experience shows both the benefits and limitations of long-term care facilities in managing schizophrenia. These facilities provide essential support and stability for residents, yet they must continually evolve to address complex and changing needs, especially concerning social interaction and becoming reintegrated into the broader community. This case study serves as a reminder of the critical need for comprehensive, individualized care for people like Michael.

Case 4. The Impact of Emily's Schizophrenia on Her Family

When Emily was formally diagnosed with schizophrenia at the age of twenty-five, the news was not just life-altering for her—it affected her entire family, changing the fabric of their lives in ways they had never anticipated. At first, Emily's family was both alarmed and bewildered by the strange and uncharacteristic behaviors she exhibited. Her once lively and engaging personality became overshadowed by bizarre symptoms that were as confusing to her as they were to those who loved her. While Emily's parents were the ones who insisted that she see a psychiatrist, even going so far as to come with her for the assessment, they were shocked when their daughter was diagnosed with schizophrenia. Like most people in their position, all that they knew about schizophrenia was what they saw in movies and television, including many of the misunderstandings and stigma surrounding the condition. Emily's family naturally found themselves grappling with the implications of her diagnosis, particularly concerning what the future might hold for her.

Before Emily's diagnosis, her family had little to no experience with mental illness, which made the situation even more daunting. Suddenly, they were thrust into a complex and often-overwhelming world of mental healthcare, one filled with medical jargon, unfamiliar treatment options, and a healthcare system that was anything but straightforward. The learning curve was steep, and they had to educate themselves rapidly to understand what schizophrenia was, what it wasn't, and how they could support Emily through the treatment process. It was a challenge to come to terms with not just the diagnosis but also the societal stigma that comes with mental illness. This stigma influenced their interactions with Emily, her healthcare providers, and community members. The fear of the unknown, compounded by their lack of experience, added another layer of stress and anxiety to an already difficult situation.

However, Emily's family's journey through her diagnosis is also a powerful illustration of the challenges and triumphs that many families face when a loved one is diagnosed with a mental health disorder. Recognizing the need to be well-informed, Emily's parents and siblings carefully educated themselves about schizophrenia. They attended support groups, sought advice from various mental health professionals, and read extensively on the subject. This dedication to learning was crucial, as it empowered them to make informed decisions about Emily's treatment and to advocate for her effectively in a healthcare system that can be notoriously difficult to navigate.

One of the most significant challenges they encountered was ensuring that Emily received the best possible care. This involved finding the right specialists and therapies that would address her specific needs. The family had to deal with the complexities of insurance coverage, which often added frustration and delays in getting Emily the treatment she needed. These bureaucratic obstacles required persistence and determination, as the family understood that getting Emily the right help was essential for her long-term well-being.

Throughout this process, the importance of family support became increasingly evident. Emily's family provided her with a stable, loving, and understanding environment, which was crucial for her to follow her treatment plan and cope with the daily challenges of schizophrenia. The support they offered was not just emotional; it was also vital in combating the stigma surrounding mental illness. By being open about Emily's condition and sharing their experiences with others, her family played a strong role in educating their community and fostering a more accepting and supportive environment. Although they faced ignorance and prejudice at times, their willingness to speak out helped to dismantle misconceptions and promote a more inclusive approach to mental health.

Emily's story is a testament to the vital role that family support plays in managing mental health disorders like schizophrenia. The emotional and practical challenges are immense, but the strength and resilience that families can develop in the face of such adversity are equally profound. Strong family support not only helps individuals like Emily to cope with the complexities of their symptoms but also positions families as powerful advocates for better mental healthcare within their communities. Stories like Emily's shed light on the individual struggles faced by those with schizophrenia and the incredible strength that families can muster when dealing with mental health challenges.

Analysis

Emily's family experience following her schizophrenia diagnosis demonstrates the profound impact mental illness has not just on individuals, but on their families as well. Though they had trouble accepting her diagnosis at first, Emily's parents and siblings quickly realized that supporting Emily meant learning as much about schizophrenia as possible, including the role they would be playing in helping her navigate the healthcare system on her behalf. Finding appropriate care required them to become advocates for Emily as she battled through insurance issues and the various mental health services available to her. This aspect of their journey highlights a common struggle many families face: the difficulty in accessing adequate mental healthcare and dealing with bureaucratic obstacles they face along the way.

In Emily's case, the unwavering support of her family provided her with a stable environment essential for her treatment and well-being. Their support meant not only supporting Emily in her day-to-day life but in working to combat the stigma associated with mental illness within their community. Not only did this make life easier for Emily, but it also promoted a broader understanding and acceptance for everyone dealing with serious mental illness.

Being diagnosed with schizophrenia represents a major challenge for patients as well as their families. It also emphasizes the importance of education, advocacy, and community engagement in navigating mental health challenges, as well as showing the vital role of family support in achieving successful management of mental health conditions.

Case 5. Liam Has Schizoaffective Disorder

Liam was thirty years old when he first began to notice that something wasn't right in his life. It wasn't just the occasional bout of sadness that troubled him; it was an overwhelming, persistent sadness that would engulf him without any apparent reason. Alongside his emotional upsets, he started developing strange, bizarre beliefs—thoughts that he knew, deep down, were irrational, yet they stubbornly clung to his mind. At first, Liam managed to keep these troubling symptoms hidden from those around him, maintaining a semblance of normalcy. But as time passed, these symptoms started to seep into his daily life, making it harder and harder for him to function.

Desperate to understand what was happening to him, Liam turned to books and online resources, trying to educate himself about mental illness. But the symptoms he experienced didn't seem to fit neatly into any of the categories he read about. This only added to his confusion and fear. Eventually, he sought professional help, making repeated visits to hospital emergency departments in hopes of finding answers. Despite his efforts, the process was anything but straightforward. The lack of a clear diagnosis left him feeling isolated and uncertain, as he struggled to make sense of his own mind.

Initially, Liam's doctors believed he was suffering from severe depression, given the intense sadness he often felt. Depression, after all, is a common diagnosis, and his mood swings seemed to fit the pattern. However, as time went on, his symptoms evolved in a way that didn't quite match typical depression. He began to experience more pronounced psychotic symptoms—delusions, hallucinations, and thoughts that were clearly detached from reality. It was then that his doctors realized something more complex was at play.

After further evaluations, Liam was finally diagnosed with schizoaffective disorder. This diagnosis, though unfamiliar to him, brought some relief. At last, there was a name for what he was experiencing, an explanation for the seemingly disjointed symptoms that had plagued him. Schizoaffective disorder is a condition that combines features of both schizophrenia and mood disorders, which explained why Liam experienced both severe mood swings and psychotic episodes.

However, receiving a diagnosis was just the beginning of a new set of challenges. Schizoaffective disorder required a carefully tailored treatment plan that addressed both aspects of his condition. Liam was prescribed antipsychotic medication to help manage the delusions and hallucinations, while mood stabilizers were added to his regimen to help control the emotional highs and lows. But medication alone wasn't enough. Liam also began attending therapy sessions, where he could talk openly about his experiences and learn strategies to cope with his symptoms more effectively.

Managing schizoaffective disorder proved to be an ongoing struggle. The symptoms didn't always respond predictably to treatment, and Liam's doctors frequently had to adjust his medications. Each adjustment brought a new set of challenges, as Liam had to contend with side effects ranging from drowsiness to weight gain. These side effects sometimes felt just as upsetting as the symptoms they were meant to treat. But through it all, Liam remained determined to regain control over his life. The gradual stability that his medications provided encouraged him to stick with his treatment plan, despite the hurdles.

Over time, Liam began to notice significant improvements in his condition. The psychotic symptoms became less frequent and less intense, and his mood swings began to level out. He also developed a better understanding of his disorder, learning to recognize the early warning signs of an impending episode. This awareness made the episodes seem less unpredictable and easier to manage, which, in turn, reduced his anxiety about the future.

Therapy played a crucial role in Liam's recovery. Both individual and group therapy sessions helped him rebuild his self-esteem, which had taken a hit during the darkest days of his illness. These sessions provided a safe space for him to express his fears and frustrations and to connect with others who were going through similar experiences. The support he found in therapy was invaluable, giving him the strength to face his challenges with resilience and hope.

As Liam's symptoms became more manageable, he felt a growing desire to help others who were facing similar struggles. He began to share his story, hoping that his experiences could offer some comfort and encouragement to those battling mental illness. Liam became an advocate for mental health awareness, speaking openly about the realities of living with schizoaffective disorder. He aimed to educate others about the condition and to fight the stigma that so often surrounds mental illness.

Liam's journey with schizoaffective disorder is ongoing. He knows that managing his symptoms will be a lifelong process, but he also knows that he doesn't have to face it alone. With a strong support system in place—including his healthcare providers, family, and community—Liam feels better equipped to handle the ups and downs that come with his condition. His story underscores the importance of personalized treatment plans and the power of resilience in the face of adversity. But perhaps most importantly, it highlights the need for compassion and understanding, both from those who treat mental illness and from the broader community. With the right support, people like Liam can lead fulfilling lives, contributing to their communities and finding their place in the world.

Analysis

Liam's experience with schizoaffective disorder exemplifies the challenges of managing mental health conditions that include both psychotic and mood disorder symptoms. Initially mistaken for severe depression due to his emotional symptoms, Liam's worsening psychotic symptoms highlighted the need for a balanced approach to diagnosis and treatment.

Schizoaffective disorder, as illustrated by Liam's experience, blurs the lines between schizophrenia and mood disorders, requiring a careful treatment strategy. For Liam, this included being placed on antipsychotics to control his delusions and hallucinations, mood stabilizers to control mood swings, and supportive therapy to help him manage his condition. Not only did therapy help

Liam cope with his symptoms but it also allowed him to rebuild his self-esteem and develop strategies to manage daily life.

Liam's case underscores the importance of personalized and comprehensive treatment plans in managing complex psychiatric conditions. His initial misdiagnosis shows the challenges involved in accurately identifying conditions with overlapping symptoms. Effective management of schizoaffective disorder requires an integrated approach that addresses both psychotic and mood components.

Moreover, Liam's advocacy for mental health awareness highlights the value of open discussions about mental illness, which can help reduce stigma and encourage others to seek help. His story is not just about the struggles associated with schizoaffective disorder but also about the resilience and advocacy that can emerge from navigating such challenges.

Glossary

Affective Flattening: Diminished emotional expression often found in schizophrenia. Individuals displaying this kind of flattening may have a reduced ability to show emotions through facial expressions, voice tone, or body language.

Alogia: Also known as poverty of speech, alogia refers to a reduction in the amount of speech schizophrenics produce as well as the kind of ideas such speech can convey. Conversations with someone experiencing alogia might feel strained, with brief, unelaborated responses that make deep communication difficult.

Anhedonia: Defined as the loss of pleasure in activities once enjoyed. For individuals experiencing anhedonia, the motivation to engage in these activities dissipates, leading to a life that can feel empty and joyless. Anhedonia can also be seen in many mood disorders.

Avolition: This term refers to a lack of motivation or ability to initiate and persist in goal-directed activities. People experiencing avolition can have problems performing everyday tasks, ranging from personal hygiene to pursuing educational or work-related goals.

Bipolar Disorder: A mental health condition characterized by extreme mood swings, including periods of high energy and euphoria (mania) and periods of deep sadness or depression.

Blunted Affect: A reduced or dull emotional response, where a person shows little or no reaction to emotional situations, even when they might normally be expected to.

Capgras Syndrome: A condition where a person believes that someone close to them, like a family member or friend, has been replaced by an identical impostor.

Catatonic Schizophrenia: This rare form of schizophrenia involves disturbances in movement. Affected individuals may exhibit motor immobility or excessive, pointless activity. Catatonia can also present with *waxy flexibility*, where an individual's limbs remain in the position they are placed by someone else, e.g., placing an arm in front of the face.

Circumstantiality: A negative symptom of schizophrenia in which someone includes excessive and unnecessary details before eventually getting to the main point.

Cognitive-Behavioral Therapy (CBT): A type of talk therapy that helps people change negative thought patterns and behaviors by focusing on the relationship between their thoughts, feelings, and actions.

Cognitive Schizophrenia Symptoms: Cognitive symptoms involve changes in memory or other aspects of thinking, like trouble focusing or following conversations, which can make everyday tasks challenging.

Cotard's Syndrome: A rare mental condition where a person believes they are dead, don't exist, or have lost their organs or blood.

Default Mode Network (DMN): A brain network thought to be involved in self-referential thoughts and the resting state. Consisting of the dorsal medial prefrontal cortex, posterior cingulate cortex, precuneus and angular gyrus, the DMN is most active during activities such as daydreaming, planning for the future, or remembering the past.

Delusional Disorder: A condition characterized by strong beliefs in things that are not real or true but don't typically feature the full spectrum of psychotic symptoms found in schizophrenia, i.e., hallucinations.

Delusions: A profound distortion of reality, where the affected person holds strong beliefs in things that are not true or highly exaggerated despite evidence. Unlike simple misbeliefs that can be corrected with new information, delusions are rigid and persist even when faced with clear evidence that contradicts them. See individual delusions listings.

Delusions of Reference: Believing that ordinary events or objects have special personal meaning or are directly related to you, even though they're not.

Dialectical Behavior Therapy (DBT): A type of therapy that combines cognitive-behavioral techniques with concepts like mindfulness and acceptance, often used to help people manage intense emotions and improve relationships.

Disorganized Schizophrenia: This type is characterized by disorganized speech and behavior, as well as flat or inappropriate emotions. Disorganized schizophrenics might have trouble organizing their thoughts or may speak in a way that's hard to understand. They may also exhibit behaviors that don't make sense or are not appropriate to the situation.

Dopamine: A neuromodulatory molecule that is the most common neurotransmitter in the human body. Along with multiple other roles, dopamine is associated with the brain's reward system and is believed to play a role in the development of psychotic symptoms.

Extrapyramidal Symptoms: Symptoms which can arise in people being treated with anti-psychotic medications. These include *dystonia* (painful muscle spasms), *akathisia* (restlessness), and *parkinsonism* (characterized by tremors, stiffness, and movement slowing). While these symptoms are largely manageable, first-generation antipsychotics can also lead to more serious conditions such as *tardive dyskinesia*, a condition marked by involuntary movements, a reminder of the medication's presence long after the day's dose, and even *neuroleptic malignant syndrome*, which can be life-threatening unless the medication is stopped immediately.

Fregoli Syndrome: A rare condition where a person believes that different people they encounter are actually the same person in disguise or changing appearances.

Glutamate: The most abundant neurotransmitter in the human body, glutamate is critical for brain plasticity and learning. As with dopamine, glutamate imbalances can disrupt the brain's normal signaling, leading to the cognitive, emotional, and behavioral symptoms characteristic of schizophrenia.

Hallucinations: Experiencing something that isn't actually there, like hearing voices or seeing things that don't exist, even though it feels real to the person.

Negative Schizophrenia Symptoms: Negative symptoms involve a diminishing or absence of the ability to function normally, such as a lack of motivation, withdrawal from social life, communication difficulties, or diminished emotional expression.

Paranoid Delusions: A false belief that others are out to harm or deceive you, even when there's no real evidence to support it.

Paranoid Schizophrenia: Once considered the most common type, individuals with this form primarily experience auditory hallucinations and delusions. For example, they might hear voices that comment on their behavior or converse with each other. They may also have delusions of persecution or grandeur, but their cognitive functions might remain relatively intact.

Personality Disorders: Defined by the Diagnostic and Statistical Manual of Mental Illness (DSM-5) as long-lasting, disruptive patterns of thinking, behavior, mood, or social functioning which can cause long-term adjustment problems for many people. Of the ten formally recognized personality disorders, schizoid, schizotypal, and paranoid personality disorders are most often confused with schizophrenia.

Polygenic Disorder: A disorder influenced by many different genes, each making a small but important contribution. Schizophrenia is believed to be one example of this.

Positive Schizophrenia Symptoms: Positive symptoms include hallucinations (seeing or hearing things that are not present) and delusions (false beliefs not based on reality), which add to one's experience of the world in a way that is not based on reality.

Psychosis: A condition of the mind that results in difficulty telling what is real from what is not, psychosis can encompass a range of symptoms, including hallucinations and impairments in reality testing.

Residual Schizophrenia: In this form, the individual might have a history of acute schizophrenia, but currently has no prominent positive symptoms (such as hallucinations or delusions). They might, however, still display negative symptoms, like withdrawal from social activities or lack of motivation. This is the form of schizophrenia most commonly seen in long-term psychiatric patients.

Schizoaffective Disorder: A mental health condition that includes symptoms of both schizophrenia (like hallucinations or delusions) and mood disorders (like depression or mania).

Somatic Delusions: A false belief that something is wrong with your body, like thinking you're sick or deformed, even though there's no medical reason for it.

Stereotyped Movements: Repetitive, purposeless movements or actions that are performed in the same way over and over, often seen in certain neurological or psychiatric conditions. It can also be a negative symptom of schizophrenia.

Tangential Speech: A negative symptom of schizophrenia involving speech that goes off on unrelated topics and never actually answers the original question or completes the main idea.

Undifferentiated Schizophrenia: This classification is used when symptoms don't clearly align with the specific types of schizophrenia but the diagnosis of schizophrenia is still appropriate. Individuals might have symptoms across different categories, making it hard to pinpoint a more specific type.

Directory of Resources

This section provides a list of resources aimed at supporting individuals with schizophrenia as well as their therapists, caregivers, family members, and friends. Each category includes tools and platforms that can be instrumental in understanding, managing, and living with schizophrenia.

Books

The Center Cannot Hold: My Journey through Madness by Elyn R. Saks, 2008

An autobiographical account of living with schizophrenia, offering insights into the personal struggles and triumphs faced by those with the condition.

Cognitive-behavioral Therapy for Schizophrenia by Gillian Haddock and Douglas Turkington, 2005

A book for therapists offering detailed approaches and techniques for treating schizophrenia using cognitive-behavioral therapy.

I Am Not Sick, I Don't Need Help! How to Help Someone with Mental Illness Accept Treatment by Xavier Amador, 2007

Useful for caregivers and family members, this book provides strategies for communicating with loved ones who are in denial about their mental illness.

Schizophrenia for Dummies by Jerome Levine and Irene S. Levine, 2008

A straightforward, easy-to-understand guide that explains the complex world of schizophrenia to patients and their families.

Surviving Schizophrenia: A Family Manual by E. Fuller Torrey, 2013

This book is a comprehensive guide that provides essential information on the nature, causes, treatment, and management of schizophrenia. It serves as a crucial resource for families and caregivers.

Hotlines

Mental Health Emergency Hotline – 988

National Alliance on Mental Illness (NAMI) HelpLine – 1-800-950-NAMI (6264) or text "HELPLINE" to 62640

National Mental Health Hotline – 1-866-903-3787
National Suicide Prevention Lifeline – 1-800-273-TALK (8255)

Online Resources

American Psychiatric Association (APA) – https://www.mhanational.org

Resources include training webinars, latest research findings, and guidelines for the treatment of schizophrenia.

Brain & Behavior Research Foundation – https://bbrfoundation.org

Shares the latest research updates and insights into mental health conditions, including schizophrenia.

Caregiver Action Network – https://www.caregiveraction.org

Provides tips and tools for caregivers of people with mental illness, including support networks.

Family Caregiver Alliance – https://www.caregiver.org

The National Center on Caregiving offers education, support, and resources tailored for the needs of family caregivers.

International Society for Psychological and Social Approaches to Psychosis (ISPS) – https://isps.org

Offers conferences and training on psychotherapy techniques for psychosis.

Mental Health America – https://www.mhanational.org

Features toolkits for self-help and information on finding professional help.

National Alliance on Mental Illness (NAMI) – https://www.nami.org

Offers information on support groups, educational programs, and local resources.

National Alliance on Mental Illness (NAMI) Family-to-Family – https://www.nami.org/support-education/mental-health-education/nami-family-to-family

A free, 8-session educational program for family, significant others, and friends of people with mental health conditions.

Psych Central – https://psychcentral.com

Provides a wealth of articles, blogs, and forums where individuals can learn about schizophrenia and discuss their experiences and coping strategies with peers.

Psychology Today – https://www.psychologytoday.com

A platform to find seminars, continuing education opportunities, and articles on current practices in schizophrenia management

Rethink Mental Illness – https://www.rethink.org

A UK-based website that offers advice, community stories, and practical support for everyone affected by schizophrenia and other mental health disorders.

SAMHSA (Substance Abuse and Mental Health Services Administration) – https://www.samhsa.gov

Offers publications and data on co-occurring disorders and holistic approaches to treatment.

SARDAA Family Toolkit – https://rootscollaborative.com/wp-content/uploads/2021/02/SARDAA-Family-Toolkit.pdf

This pamphlet from the Schizophrenia & Psychosis Action Alliance (formerly known as SARDAA) offers guidance on how family members can support a loved one with schizophrenia.

SchizLife – https://www.schizlife.com

A site dedicated to providing a deep understanding of schizophrenia from a personal perspective. It includes coping strategies, daily life tips, and extensive background on the condition.

Schizophrenia.com – http://schizophrenia.com

A comprehensive site offering forums, treatment options, and research updates to individuals, families, and healthcare providers.

Schizophrenia: World Health Organization – https://www.who.int/news-room/fact-sheets/detail/schizophrenia

Offers wide range of resources on schizophrenia from around the world. It also covers comprehensive information on mental health initiatives by the WHO.

Schizophrenia and Related Disorders Alliance of America (SARDAA) – https://sczaction.org/sardaa

Provides assistance through programs like Schizophrenics Anonymous, a self-help group.

StrengthofUs.org – https://youth.gov/shared-resources/strengthofusorg-live-better-life-through-community

An online community developed by the National Alliance on Mental Illness (NAM) that offers resources and support specifically for young adult caregivers.

Index

About the Author

Romeo Vitelli received his doctorate in psychology from York University in Toronto, Ontario, in 1987 and has been in private practice since 2003. His published works with ABC-CLIO/Bloomsbury include *Autism: Your Questions Answered* (2023), *What You Need to Know about Schizophrenia* (2021), *Depression: Your Questions Answered* (2019), *Self-Injury: Your Questions Answered* (2018), and *Substance Abuse: Your Questions Answered* (2018).